# WHAT DID I JUST EAT?
## *Surprising Facts About Food!*

By Dr. Patrick Baker, Dr. Paul Baker and Dr. Ryan Berlin

Cover Design by Amber Miller.

©Copyright 2011

# WHAT DID I JUST EAT?
*Surprising Facts About Food!*

By Dr. Patrick Baker, Dr. Paul Baker and Dr. Ryan Berlin

**©Copyright 2011 by Dr. Paul Baker and Dr. Patrick Baker.**

Printed in the United States of America

First Printing, 2011

For permission to reproduce, and to order additional copies of this book,
contact: Baker Chiropractic and Wellness, (513) 561-2273.

# TABLE OF CONTENTS

PREFACE

## INTRODUCTION
*The Most Important Nutrition Principle: Nutrient Density*

## PART ONE...**THE BAD STUFF**

## PART TWO...**THE GOOD STUFF**

**REFERENCES**

# PREFACE

## *The Start of a Better Life*

We all look for ways to improve our life. As a result, we are constantly bombarded with a wide variety of products and services that make all kinds of promises to make life better. Simply Google the keyword phrase "improve your life," and you will find everything from convenient electronic devices to medications claiming to treat nearly every type of health condition to thousands of diet and exercise plans for losing weight.

The reality of it all is there is no one single magic "bullet" for improving your life. However, there are some fundamentals that create a solid foundation to realize your true potential for a life filled with health, happiness and satisfaction.

The three of us (Dr. Paul Baker, Dr. Patrick Baker and Dr. Ryan Berlin) were given precious gifts early in life. We all suffered from different health conditions at very young ages, which medications and even surgery failed to correct. Like all good parents, our mothers and fathers continued to look for answers.

They found those answers in chiropractic care and the power of the human body. Once relieved of our problematic health conditions, each of us found a strong respect and admiration for taking care of our bodies. We adopted principles of health and wellness and incorporated those principles into every fabric of our lives. It has rewarded us greatly in our personal and our professional lives. Our experience became the driving force that motivated us to become physicians and provide others with the gift of health and happiness through education, inspiration and high quality chiropractic care.

We are all graduates of the prestigious Palmer Chiropractic College located in Davenport, Iowa. The chiropractic practice has been widely viewed as a radical alternative to traditional medical care since Palmer Chiropractic College was founded in 1895. However, nothing could be further from the truth.

A Doctor of Chiropractic (D.C.) must obtain a formal education that is very similar to a medical doctor's education. In fact, chiropractic colleges have the same admission requirements as medical schools. They dictate diverse undergraduate studies focused on science, biology, chemistry, anatomy and physics. When enrolled in a chiropractic college, students must complete four to five years of extensive study and training to earn their Doctorate of Chiropractic.

The first two years of chiropractic and medical school are alike. After these first two years, the distinctions start to emerge. Medical students begin their focus on pharmacology (drugs), critical care and surgery. Chiropractic students partake in intense studies of the central nervous system, the causes and effects of subluxations and the human body's ability to heal and restore itself.

Doctors of Chiropractic are regulated just like the medical professional. They must obtain a license from the state in which they practice after passing multi-day National Board Examinations as well as additional testing requirements imposed by many states. Each state also has annual continuing education requirements that Doctors of Chiropractic must complete to maintain their state license.

The scientific community has taken note of the effectiveness of the chiropractic profession over the past 30 years. There is an abundance of information on numerous research studies conducted on the results and benefits derived from routine chiropractic care and proper nutrition.

Our approach to healthcare is to utilize chiropractic care, wellness principles (like diet and exercise) and medical care, in that order. We serve as the primary care physician for many of our patients. This saves our patients significant time and money. It's a very logical and common sense approach that allows your body to perform as it is designed.

The human body is equipped with a very powerful immune system that fights disorders, diseases, viruses and bacteria better than any prescription medication. When your body is optimized and permitted to fully function, it will prevent itself from being overrun by toxins, viruses and bacteria that evolve into overwhelming health problems. This is achieved through the proper blend of nutritional intake, chiropractic care, fitness and general knowledge of your body.

It's not our intention to discount the importance of medical care. There are traumatic events in people's lives requiring emergency medical care. The advanced stages of disease also necessitate the assistance of medical specialists and skilled surgeons to save lives. When medical care is required, there will be a recovery period. Chiropractic care and professional guidance on proper nutrition, avoiding toxins and reducing stress greatly enhances and improves healing times and the return of normal function. As primary care physicians, we create a chiropractic and medical alliance that serves the best interest of our patients with their physical health and their financial health.

The starting point for a life of health and happiness is the food we eat. You can and will change the way you look and the way you feel simply by giving your body the proper food at the right times. Most of us do not really know what we are putting in our mouths and our bodies. We are influenced by marketing messages from food companies that want us to buy their products. Many of these companies attempt to compel our consumption of their products by insinuating their products are good for us.

Our society has also been saturated with virtually every conceivable diet plan telling us to count calories, reduce food portions or eat only specially prepared food. These are just a few examples of the misinformation and misconceptions about the food we eat. Once you understand what you are eating, it's easy to make decisions and choices about food. Choices that will help you lose weight, increase energy and help your body reach a new level of health.

Rather than concerning ourselves with how many calories we are eating, we should be focused on the nutrient levels contained within the food. The typical diet of an American is filled with foods that are nutrient poor. Therefore, our bodies demand and crave more food in order to get the amount of nutrients needed to function properly. We also live with traditions and a culture of eating a very light breakfast, then increasing our food intake at lunch and culminating the day with a very large dinner. The proper way of consuming food is the exact opposite. We should start with a large, nutrient-rich breakfast and reduce our food intake over the course of the day while staying focused on providing our bodies with nutrient-rich foods.

In the chapters and pages that follow, we look at the low-nutrient foods you need to avoid and foods you may have been deceived into falsely believing are "healthy." We provide you with countless options for healthy foods that are not only tasty but full of nutrients. We also reveal foods you thought were unhealthy that actually help you!

We dig into the truth about cholesterol, saturated fats, omega 3s and omega 6s, fiber, protein, hormones, plant foods vs. animal foods, and tons of information that may shock you about what's in the food you buy at grocery stores and restaurants.

The food you give your body is the starting point for a life of health and happiness. We hope this book provides you with the education and the stimulation to take a hard look at your eating habits and the food you are consuming on a daily basis. We hope it also provides the motivation to start taking more control of your life by making the changes that will lead to health and happiness.

After reading our book, we invite you to visit our website at www. doctorspaulandpatrick.com to learn more about us. While visiting our website, please send your questions or arrange for a personal and private telephone consultation directly with us. We would be delighted and honored to help you start living a healthier and happier life.

In Health,

*Dr. Paul Baker, Dr. Patrick Baker and Dr. Ryan Berlin*

# INTRODUCTION

## *The Most Important Nutrition Principle: Nutrient Density*

The most important thing you can measure is the nutrient density of your food intake.

Stop counting calories! Calories consumed versus calories expended over a specific time period is what ultimately controls whether you gain weight or lose weight.

However, not only is counting calories horribly inaccurate (studies show that the majority of people massively underestimate their caloric intake when asked to count calories), but calorie counting is pointless once you understand the most important nutrition principle: nutrient density.

Nutrient density makes calorie counting obsolete. If all of the foods you eat every day are comprised of super-high micro-nutrient density, then your body obtains all of the nutrition it needs and automatically regulates your appetite and calorie intake.

Nutrient-dense food includes more than just fruits and vegetables. Throughout this book you'll find that high nutrient density can also include lots of fatty foods that you may have wrongly been taught should be eliminated, such as whole eggs, certain types of meats, nuts, nut butters, certain oils, butter, and so on.

If you eat foods each day that are high in calories but low in nutrients - such as pasta, cakes, cookies and crackers (high caloric density, low nutrient density) - then your body will be craving additional food. You may have already eaten more than the allotted amount of calories that day to maintain your weight, but you'll still be hungry.

On the other hand, if all of the foods you eat on a daily basis are high in nutrient density, regardless of the caloric content of those foods, your body will adjust your appetite and eliminate cravings based on already having obtained much of the nutrition it needs for the day. This aspect essentially forces your body to "auto-adjust" your appetite, and you naturally fall within the exact calorie range that your body needs without having to over-analyze or count calories.

In fact, eating a super-high nutrient dense diet is so powerful that extreme distance athletes, who burn massive amounts of calories each day through excessive exercise, may actually need to focus on consuming a portion of their diet as lower nutrient density foods, such as breads, pasta and other calorically-dense but low-nutrient foods, to avoid massive weight loss. The reason for this is that if an extreme distance athlete focuses too much of their diet on super-high nutrient density foods, their appetite may be diminished before they actually have eaten enough calories to sustain their massive calorie needs, and excessive weight loss may occur.

Since most of us are not extreme distance athletes, this just shows you the power of eating a super-high nutrient dense diet, and how this can automatically control your appetite, eliminate cravings and put you on the road to a lean, healthy body for life.

# 1 The First Step

*Start the Kitchen Cleanout!*

Here's a typical list of "food" that the average person trying to lose weight may have on hand. Check your cabinets and see if any of this fat fuel is lurking in your kitchen:

*Slim-Fast® shakes* - Far from healthy, they're actually loaded with high-fructose corn syrup, hydrogenated oils and a bunch of other chemicals that will add fat to your body, not aid in weight loss.

*Fat-free rice cakes* - These really are nothing but pure, refined starch with zero fiber, which breaks down immediately into sugar in your body, spiking insulin and promoting fat storage.

*Protein/energy bars* – A combination of isolated soy protein (virtually unusable by your body), hydrogenated oils, high-fructose corn syrup and artificial preservatives, these are basically a candy bar in a deceiving package. Toss quickly into the nearest trash can!

*Reduced sugar desserts* –A mad scientist's experiment gone awry, such desserts are loaded with artificial sweeteners (that trick your brain and trigger hunger), sugar alcohols, preservatives, and a chemical ingredient list about 15 lines long. Nothing at all good in there.

*Diet soda* - Loaded with artificial sweeteners like NutraSweet® or Splenda® that do more harm than good, raise the insulin levels in your body and cause you to be hungry and store fat. Diet? We hardly think so!

*Chips, crackers and cookies*- Loaded with hydrogenated (read "heart attack in a box") fats, inflammatory processed omega-6 oils, and processed flours. High- carb foods that add weight almost instantly!

*Refined vegetable oils* - Canola oil, corn oil, soybean oil, sunflower oil, safflower oil, Crisco and the like, used for cooking and salad dressings, are composed mostly of oxidized omega-6 fatty acids, which lead to inflammation, heart disease, weight gain and fat around the midsection.

*Sugary cereals*- Advertised as healthy and high fiber, these cereals are loaded with sugar and refined fat-factory grains such as corn, soybean flour and wheat. They will make you hungrier, spike your blood sugar and increase your insulin response, thus putting your body into a fat-storing mode.

# THE HEALTHY EATING PYRAMID

Most of us are familiar with the USDA's Food Guide Pyramid from our school years. It was introduced by the U.S. Department of Agriculture (USDA) many years ago to teach the public about nutrition. However, it touts a low-fat, high-carbohydrate diet, which is contradictory to most of today's healthy eating messages from doctors, nutritionists and the like. It also does not distinguish between good fats and bad fats nor does it differentiate between the different kinds of grains, meat and dairy products – some of which are a necessary part of a healthy, daily diet, while others just add pounds.

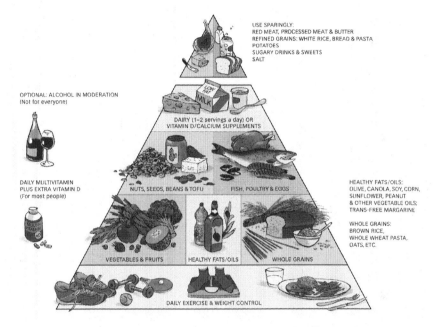

USE SPARINGLY:
RED MEAT, PROCESSED MEAT & BUTTER
REFINED GRAINS: WHITE RICE, BREAD & PASTA
POTATOES
SUGARY DRINKS & SWEETS
SALT

OPTIONAL: ALCOHOL IN MODERATION
(Not for everyone)

DAIRY (1–2 servings a day) OR
VITAMIN D/CALCIUM SUPPLEMENTS

DAILY MULTIVITAMIN
PLUS EXTRA VITAMIN D
(For most people)

NUTS, SEEDS, BEANS & TOFU    FISH, POULTRY & EGGS

HEALTHY FATS/OILS:
OLIVE, CANOLA, SOY, CORN,
SUNFLOWER, PEANUT
& OTHER VEGETABLE OILS;
TRANS-FREE MARGARINE

WHOLE GRAINS:
BROWN RICE,
WHOLE WHEAT PASTA,
OATS, ETC.

VEGETABLES & FRUITS    HEALTHY FATS/OILS    WHOLE GRAINS

DAILY EXERCISE & WEIGHT CONTROL

Thanks to the Harvard School of Public Health's Healthy Eating Pyramid (pictured above), we can put aside confusions such as whether to eat more fats and less carbs, or no carbs and more protein. The Harvard Healthy Eating Pyramid shows us that good nutrition is not just about fat vs. carbs, but rather is built on a base of daily exercise and weight control. Each block has been re-structured from the bottom up to show the most important elements of a healthy diet and how much of each element we should intake each day.

Initially, you should consult your doctor to find out the appropriate weight for your height and body structure, and what types of exercise he or she recommends for you. From there, the Harvard Healthy Eating Pyramid can be a helpful tool on your journey to changing what and how you eat and becoming the healthiest YOU you can be!

# 2 The Processing of Foods

*It is the processing of foods that truly controls how our bodies react to the food we eat.*

With all of the macronutrient debate in recent years over what type of "diet" is best for us (low-carb, low-fat, no-carb, high protein, vegetarian, etc.), you've got to realize that they are *all wrong!* That's right... If you study historical dietary patterns of ancestral humans in almost any culture around the world, the one aspect in common that accounted for the health benefits in each culture was that foods were unprocessed, natural foods.

Whether a diet was high in protein, high in fat, high in carbs, low in carbs, etc., didn't seem to matter that much as long as the diet was made up of natural, unprocessed foods eaten as close as possible to how they were found in nature.

We gain weight and get fat when more calories are eaten on a regular basis than our bodies need to meet daily energy demands. When excess calories get stored as fat, it is the body's way of answering in a revolutionary response from the hunter-gatherer days when food was less plentiful and people had to put out a great effort just to survive.

Way back when, people who were able to store food in the form of fat were more likely to survive and reproduce during times of scarcity. Because of this advantage, we still have that innate urge to eat a lot of food when it is available, and some more than others. And there is a lot of food - or junk - that is available to us everywhere we turn these days!

In spite of being able to store body fat efficiently, ancestral humans were rarely obese because they had to work hard just to eat, and in the process burned up whatever calories they consumed.

The huge agricultural and technological changes of the past two thousand years have made food extremely easy to obtain, and evolution has not been able to keep pace in the short time span. We no longer have to spend our days hunting and searching out food; there is an abundance everywhere we look.

While the reasons we gain weight are numerous, there are some primary reasons for the excess fat that we carry around. If we remove the food that causes fat storage, and erase a big part of the temptation to eat overly processed, fattening foods, we should be on our way to transforming our bodies into lean, energetic machines.

Not only will we see stronger, leaner bodies, but many of the modern diseases will begin to fade away: irritability, depression, ADD, arthritis, high blood sugar/Type 2 diabetes, irritable bowel syndrome, and on and on. All are connected to inflammation and the Standard American Diet (S.A.D.) of processed junk.

We have been duped into believing that instant, fast, pre-made foods will somehow make us thin and healthy. If you check out your grocery store's frozen food aisle, you will often see overweight people purchasing what they think are "diet dinners." Nothing could be further from the truth! Processed "diet" dinners are chock full of preservatives, high-fructose corn syrup, processed flours, synthetic fillers, soy protein, and the worst kind of fats. These foods will cause inflammation, stimulate the insulin response (i.e., store fat) and do nothing for you nutritionally. What's more, you will GAIN weight from eating this kind of junk!

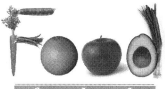

The media has fooled us into thinking we need lots and lots of carbohydrates, by standards of the U.S.D.A. Food Pyramid. In response, America has loaded up on the processed carbs and packed on the pounds. Even so-called "health foods" are often not what our bodies recognize as good nutrition or fuel. And forget fat-free (loaded with sugar and starchy carbs instead) and sugar-free! This stuff is poison and fat storing fuel.

*Our bodies, since the days of cavemen, were made to function best on whole, unprocessed foods, good quality proteins, healthy fats, and fruits and vegetables. If we can get back to a diet as close as possible to our ancestors, we will have the lean, strong bodies that we strive for.*

Forget fast and convenient diet foods! They take years off your life by stoking the fires of inflammation, which leads to such diseases as obesity, heart disease, cancer and diabetes, in addition to messing up your body's metabolism and making it increasingly difficult to lose fat from your frame. If you want healthy and clean "diet food," pick up a raw apple, some unprocessed nuts, some nitrate and corn syrup-free, grass-fed beef jerky, and nibble away to your heart's content. We need to get back to REAL food and eating like our lean, strong ancestors.

# 3 The Truth About Refined Flour and Grains

*Pasta, cookies, crackers and bread*

C ave men didn't eat grains, at least nowhere close to the form we eat today. It's no wonder then that grains are responsible for weight gain and high blood sugar. In the 1970s, the average American ate 85 pounds of flour, 84 pounds of sweeteners, 8 pounds of fried potatoes, and 39 pounds of cooking oil per year.

By 1997, each of us was consuming 122 pounds of flour, 105 pounds of sugar or other sweeteners, 20 pounds of fried potatoes, and 50 pounds of vegetable cooking oils a year. That's almost a pound of knowingly bad-for-you foods per day, and that doesn't count a whole lot of other junk food. Today, flours are more refined than ever, missing fiber and essential nutrients.

All of this clearly points to the main reason many people are overweight or obese.

Processed white flour (alias "enriched wheat flour" or "wheat flour") is missing the two most nutritious and fiber-rich parts of the seed: the outside bran layer and the germ (embryo).

Eating a high starch diet will make you feel fatigued, malnourished, constipated, jumpy, irritable, depressed, and vulnerable to chronic illness. And, refined/bleached wheat and corn flour fuels high blood sugar levels. High blood sugar leads to insulin release, immediate fat storage and further hunger.

The more refined foods a person eats, the more insulin must be produced to manage it. This leads to insulin resistance, Type 2 diabetes and weight gain. The refined carbohydrates turn to glucose very quickly once in our systems, stimulating the body to produce insulin. A vicious cycle occurs: insulin promotes the storage of fat, making way for rapid weight gain and elevated triglyceride levels, inflammation and atherosclerosis, Type 2 diabetes, and heart disease.

"Enriched flour" is very misleading because only four vitamins and minerals are typically added back, compared to the 15 nutrients and essential parts of the grain that are removed along with most of the fiber and other beneficial substances such as antioxidants.

Eating wheat can cause one to feel lethargic, foggy, groggy, puffy, bloated and irritable. Many would never connect these symptoms with eating grains, but weight gain, emotional, physical and mental symptoms are fairly frequent with gluten sensitivity. Gluten is the protein portion of wheat, rye and barley. It is so widespread in standard processed food today that it is very hard to escape. Unfortunately, gluten sensitivity is on the rise (notice the "gluten free" sections at the grocery store?) and it can cause a host of problems. Best to avoid processed flours altogether!

The American food supply is also heavily based on corn. Bumper crops of corn help to keep corn prices low, which in turn helps to keep many of the items we buy at the store low-priced.

Contrary to popular belief, corn is a grain, not a vegetable, and is really not appropriate as a dietary staple for several reasons—one of them being that corn has a high sugar content. When civilizations such as the Mayans and Native Americans changed their diet to a corn- based one, rates of anemia, arthritis, rickets and osteoporosis skyrocketed.

Our bodies were not made to exist on grain-based foods. This evidence shows up in the archeological records of our ancestors. When archaeologists looked at skeletons of native Americans in burial mounds in the Midwest who ate corn as their primary staple, there was a 50 percent increase in malnutrition, four times as much incidence of iron-deficiency, and three times as much infectious disease, compared to the more hunter-gatherer ancestors who primarily hunted and did not eat grain.

Keep in mind that we are not just talking about corn-on-the-cob (sweet corn) here... we are also talking about corn cereals, corn chips and other modern day corn-based foods that are promoted by food companies as "healthy." There are several reasons researchers give for the nutritional problems and the weight gain caused by a corn-dominated diet:

* Corn contains lots of sugar, which raises insulin levels, causes you to be hungrier and causes your body to store calories as fat. Don't be mistaken, just because corn does not taste obviously sweet, doesn't mean it isn't full of sugars. Once eaten, your body quickly turns corn products into sugar. Even the starches in corn products can be broken down quickly by your body spiking your blood sugar levels, and causing cravings for more carbohydrate-based foods.

* Corn also is a poor source of protein, usually deficient in three of the eight essential amino acids: lysine, isoleucine and tryptophan. The essential amino acids are so named because they must be obtained from the diet, since the body is unable to manufacture them.

* Corn contains a high amount of phytate, a chemical that binds iron and inhibits its absorption by the body. So, consequently, a diet high in phytate can make people more likely to have iron-deficiency anemia and fatigue. Phytate is also a nutrient blocker and inhibits other vitamins and minerals from being utilized.

* Corn is a poor source of certain minerals such as calcium and some vitamins such as niacin (B3). Deficiencies of niacin can result in a condition known as Pellagra, which is common in civilizations that eat a lot of corn. It can cause a variety of symptoms such as dermatitis, diarrhea, and depression. Since we are now a nation of corn-eaters, it wouldn't be surprising that this is more common here than we realize.

Humans are not the only ones who eat too much corn. A large amount of the nation's corn crop ends up feeding commercially raised cattle, which are cheaply fattened on corn and other grains before slaughter. Beef from corn-fattened cattle also has much higher ratios of inflammatory omega-6 fatty acids than healthier grass-fed beef. Most meat in supermarkets comes from grain-fed animals.

Because corn and other grains are an unnatural diet and difficult to digest, cattle raised on corn develop higher stomach acidity, which is a breeding ground for the dangerous E. coli O157:H7, the deadly strain of the bacteria.

While eliminating refined grains such as corn and wheat can seem a very daunting task (yes, it seems they are in everything!), the reward is a return to wonderful health, sparkling eyes, clear skin, clear thinking, weight loss (as the body is once again able to extract appropriate nutrients from food), and a resolution of nutritional deficiencies from the lack of absorption. Once you commit to eating a diet of whole and natural foods, you will begin to eliminate a large amount of these grains.

Although many grocery stores, health foods stores and online companies are now offering a wide selection of wheat-free/gluten-free foods

## FOODS to AVOID

### REFINED FLOURS

*White bread, rolls, buns, muffins*
*Cookies*
*Crackers*
*Enriched flour pasta*
*Cakes, cake mix*
*Cereal made with refined (instead of whole grain) flour*
*Pre-made, packaged gravies, sauces*
*Pre-packaged macaroni and cheese*
*Instant noodle cups, ramen noodles*
*Pre-made dinners with pasta*
*White flour for baking*
*Corn chips; Doritos®, Fritos®, Sun Chips®*
*Corn tortillas*
*Corn cereals especially the refined, sweetened ones*
*Anything with corn as one of the main ingredients*

including breads, bagels, cookies, cake mixes, doughnuts, etc. It is best to avoid these as much as possible. While they are made without wheat, they still contain other refined and processed grains and wheat substitutes such as tapioca flour and corn flour. Best thing to do is avoid grains - especially wheat and corn- - all together. Substituting another processed grain may bring about a small improvement, but not the drastic improvement necessary.

Try two weeks with no grain products. We guarantee you will see some drastic improvements in your weight and general outlook!

# 4 The Truth About Sugars and High-Fructose Corn Syrup

*High-fructose corn syrup is found in soda, fruit drinks, ketchup, salad dressings and more*

One of the many other uses of corn is the low-cost sweetener, high-fructose corn syrup (HFCS). Production of high-fructose corn syrup has increased some 4,000 percent since 1973, and the syrup now rivals sugar as America's most common sweetener.

Teenagers typically get 15 to 20 teaspoons per day of added sugars from HFCS — just from drinking soft drinks! One study shows that soft drinks have replaced milk as a dietary staple and have become the third-most-common breakfast food. Starting the day with a sugar high leads to a crash in about two hours, causing more hunger and weight gain. No wonder so many teens are overweight.

If the average American could cut just one soft drink or sugared water drink a day they would immediately cut out 10 pounds a year. In 2009, approximately 25 percent of the average American's caloric intake came from sugars — mostly HFCS. That's 25 percent of the diet filled with not only empty, but also harmful calories!

The next time you're at the supermarket, pick up five totally different kinds of bottled drinks — including juices and energy or sport waters — and read the labels. You may be shocked to see that the first or second ingredient will almost always be HFCS.

Now for a real education. Look at the labels of other items in which you would never expect to find any sweeteners: ketchup, tomato sauce, soup, cereal, and crackers. HFCS is everywhere; in one day it is entirely possible that 80 percent of the processed food you consume is chock full of HFCS. Is it any wonder there is so much obesity in the U.S.?

What is high fructose corn syrup? High-fructose corn syrup is not a natural product as you may have been led to believe, but is chemically altered by enzymatic processes to yield a different balance of sugars than that found in ordinary corn syrup (not that ordinary corn syrup is healthy either). That chemical alteration changes the extracted corn syrup from a compound that is mainly glucose (a simple sugar, such as table sugar) to around 42–55 percent fructose (fruit sugar), though some can range as high as 90 percent fructose. The remainder becomes glucose and other sugars.

A 2004 study reported in the *American Journal of Clinical Nutrition* cites the increase in consumption of HFCS between 1970 and 1990 to be 4,000 percent! This is way higher than any other increase of any other food or food group. Too bad we haven't increased our intake of fruits and vegetables by that amount. Our country would be in far better health — and much slimmer!

In studying this increase — and the nearly equivalent increase in obesity in the U.S. — these researchers took into account the differences in the way the body responds to different types of sugars and their effects on the body.

### *Fructose is converted to fat in the body more easily than any other sugar.*

There is a difference between how fructose and glucose are metabolized in the body. Glucose enters the cells through the action of insulin; fructose enters the cells through a totally separate action, which does not depend on insulin. The result is a rise in blood sugar, followed by a rise in insulin.

Fructose is not easily digested, either. Once inside the cells, fructose forms triglycerides ( a major factor in heart attacks) more efficiently than does glucose. This means that fructose will convert to fatty compounds in the blood, which are then stored easily in the body as fat.

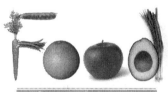

Regular sugar provides a feeling of satisfaction, which signals to the brain to stop eating. Fructose does not provide a feeling of satiety, because it is not transported into the brain.

*The average American now consumes a whopping 42 pounds of high-fructose corn syrup each year, according to U.S. Department of Agriculture data. That's an extra 75,281 calories per year, per person! If you look at that in terms of pounds (approx. 3500 calories = 1 pound), you are looking at gaining an extra 22 pounds a year.*

When fructose and glucose are found in nature (such as in apples or honey) they are typically found partnered with enzymes or fiber, which slows down the rate at which they are absorbed and utilized in the body. This slower rate negates any of their harmful effects and maximizes their healthy effects.

It seems very obvious that high-fructose corn syrup is largely responsible for the big jump in obesity and other obesity-related health issues, namely heart disease, insulin resistance and diabetes.

High-fructose corn syrup almost always comes from genetically-modified corn, which is full of its own well-documented side effects and health concerns.

Scientists have found that animals fed genetically-modified (GM) corn developed extensive health problems in the blood, kidneys and liver. Humans eating genetically modified corn may also be at risk for health issues.

When something is genetically modified, everything that makes it beneficial is destroyed. The gene code is altered so that it no longer does something it is supposed to do. This may make a product larger or better looking, or more juicy, but there is always a cost. Genetically altered food has been shown to disrupt our own DNA, causing health issues, reproductive problems, drastically reducing mental function, causing diseases, etc.

The reason genetically-modified food exists is two-fold. First, it produces food that has a larger yield, which means more profit for the farmer. Such food also does not reproduce, which means farmers have to buy new seed every year – they can no longer save and use seed from the previous year's yield. This means more profit for the food industry (seed suppliers).

*More than half of tested samples of HFCS contain mercury.*

Although the makers of HFCS like to claim that it's natural, HFCS is a highly refined product that would never exist in nature. Converting corn to HFCS is a very extensive process, and mercury is used in the production of the HFCS.

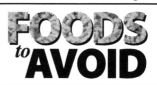

## HIGH-FRUCTOSE CORN SYRUP

*Flavored drinks or juices*
*Lemonade*
*Sports drinks like*
*    Gatorade®, etc.*
*Applesauce, fruit cocktail,*
*    canned fruits that don't say*
*    100% fruit*
*Barbeque sauces,*
*    ketchup, steak sauce*
*Alcoholic drink mixes*
*    (margarita mix, etc)*
*Puddings, Jell-O®, yogurt*
*Ice-cream products*
*Pre-made cakes, desserts*
*Kid's juice box drinks*
*Candy Cereal*
*Syrup other than pure*
*    maple syrup or no*
*    high-fructose syrups*
*Granola bars*

*Anything pre-made and pre-packaged most likely has corn syrup or HFCS in it.*

*You can avoid it if you focus your diet on whole, healthy, natural foods. If you do purchase any processed foods, make sure you read the label ... and put it back on the shelf if it lists high-fructose corn syrup as an ingredient. Keep looking. Food companies are starting to realize the general public's growing distaste for HFCS and are beginning to use sugar again, and even the natural (better for you) low-calorie sweetener, stevia.*

*Choose organic items because they do not contain high-fructose corn syrup.*

We have all heard about the dangers of ingesting mercury: it acts as a poison to your brain and nervous system. It is especially dangerous for pregnant women and small children, whose brains are still developing. Even in low doses, mercury can interfere with brain development, memory and learning ability.

In adults, mercury poisoning can be a serious risk as well, and has been linked to Alzheimer's, dementia, fertility problems, memory and vision loss, and trouble with blood pressure regulation. It can also cause extreme fatigue and neuro-muscular dysfunction.

Other studies show that mercury in your central nervous system causes psychological, neurological and immunological problems.

# 5 Processed and Diet Foods

*Preservatives, fillers, chemicals, dyes and trans fats*

There are many chemicals and flavor enhancers in processed foods and so-called "diet" foods packaged as weight-loss dinners, desserts, snacks, etc. Many of these chemicals are addictive. MSG is one good example. People who eat foods that are flavor enhanced with monosodium glutamate, or MSG, are more likely than others to be overweight or obese, even with the same amount of physical activity and caloric intake, according to the University of North Carolina at Chapel Hill School of Public Health.

Researchers at UNC and in China studied more than 750 Chinese men and women, between the ages of 40 and 59, in three rural villages in north and south China. The majority of study participants prepared their meals at home without commercially processed foods. About 82 percent of the participants used MSG in their food. Those users were divided into three groups, based on the amount of MSG they used. The group who used the most MSG was nearly three times more likely to be overweight than non-users.

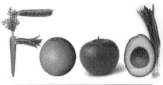

*for thought*

*The best way to avoid MSG is simply to avoid all processed foods. For some people, that may sound difficult, but it really becomes simple if the only foods that you buy at the grocery store are one-ingredient foods – that means fresh, whole, unprocessed foods.*

Because MSG is used as a flavor enhancer in many processed foods, studying its potential effect on humans has been difficult. Study participants were chosen from rural Chinese villages because they used very little commercially processed food, but many regularly used MSG in food preparation.

The bottom line is that you should avoid MSG as much as possible since it can stimulate cravings and lead to weight gain, among other problems.

Most low-calorie foods cut calories by removing refined cane sugar and replacing it with artificial sweeteners like aspartame, sucralose

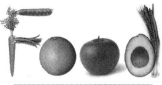

*Cravings are usually a signal your body is not getting the nutrients it needs.*

*The only certain way to lose weight permanently is to focus on healthy nutrition such as organic fruits and vegetables, raw nuts and seeds, grass-fed meats, free-range poultry and raw dairy products, an active lifestyle, reducing stress, and creating balance and harmony in our lives.*

and a dozen other sugar-like compounds. These artificial sugars contain less (in some cases, zero) calories, but they are incredibly dangerous in other ways, as we will discuss in chapter 6.

Artificial sweeteners have been linked to cancer, migraines, depression, birth defects, infertility, seizures, thyroid problems, and weight gain. Sugars and starches stimulate appetite and increase cravings for sugar—as do most artificial sweeteners.

Many nutrition experts believe that the more refined a food is, the less satisfying it is to the body. Because the body is unable to extract what it needs from denatured, highly processed junk foods, it craves more nourishment. In addition, low-calorie diet foods are usually loaded with processed ingredients that the body doesn't know what to do with, so it stores them as waste in fat stores within the body.

Among the most common processed ingredients are refined/enriched flour, colors, preservatives which go by hundreds of different names and chemical flavorings, which may legally be called "natural flavors" even if they include MSG. As a side note: most varieties of processed or "textured" soy protein (TSP or TVP) use MSG for flavor and call it "natural flavors."

Even the best food companies, whose apparent goal is to promote health and wellness, are still in business to make a profit. Corporations selling diet

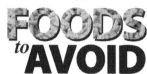

### PROCESSED FOODS

*Weight Watchers®*
*Lean Cuisine®,*
*SmartOnes®,*
*Healthy Choice®,*
*Kid Cuisine®*
*Cool Whip® Lite,*
*Cool Whip® Free,*
*Cool Whip® Sugar-free*
*Sugar-free popsicles,*
*  sugar-free ice-cream*
*Sugar-free or fat-free*
*  desserts, cookies,*
*  cakes, etc.*
*Slim Fast® shakes,*
*  bars, powder mix*
*Instant Breakfast*
*Fiber One® poptarts,*
*  cookies, muffins, etc.*
*Special K® Bars*
*Rice cakes*
*Anything packaged,*
*  processed or with*
*  the words, "low fat,"*
*  "sugar free," "fat*
*  free," "diet," etc.*

foods and low-cal foods are hardly motivated to make a product that really helps people consume less and lose weight. If they did, their captive audience - people who are overweight - would disappear, taking their money with them.

Weight loss products are highly suspect for their harmful and addictive artificial ingredients, and for the elusive promise of the "quick, easy" weight loss they promise, but almost never fulfill.

# 6 Artificial Sweeteners

*Sucralose, aspartame and saccharin*

Do diet sweeteners really help you lose weight, or do you eat more and gain weight in the long run? Do diet sweeteners make you fat? Artificial sweeteners as diet food? Hardly!

The fact is, artificial sweeteners can actually make you gain weight because they trick your body and don't feed it what it actually needs. They are chemical concoctions with NO food value that make your body think it is eating something sweet. They also contain by-products of harmful toxins, and should never be ingested!

Anyone who cares about their health should stay away from the highly toxic sweetener aspartame (NutraSweet®, Equal®) and other questionable sweeteners such as sucralose (Splenda®), saccharin (Sweet-n-Low®), and acesulfame-k (Sunette®).

According to researchers, there is no actual evidence that sugar substitutes help people lose weight. More and more, data suggests that these chemical sweeteners may actually stimulate appetite and insulin response.

How do artificial sweeteners fool the body? Aspartame, for instance, doesn't have any calories, but one of its ingredients, the amino acid phenylalanine, blocks production of serotonin, a natural brain chemical that, among other things, controls food cravings.

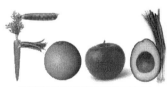

When you have a shortage of serotonin in the brain, it will make your brain and body crave the foods that create more of this brain chemical—and those happen to be the starchy, high-calorie, carbohydrate-rich snacks that can totally sabotage a diet. As you increase the amount of aspartame you take in, the more intense your cravings for these foods.

Scientists now suspect that something

*Artificial sweeteners confuse the body and brain. This leads to a vicious cycle of cravings, eating more, using more artificial sweeteners, and more cravings. Long term, you are looking at weight gain as the primary result.*

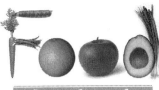

*Did you know that saccharin (also known as benzoic sulfinide or E954) was discovered in 1879 by a chemist researching coal tar derivatives? Think of this the next time you grab that little pink package to sweeten your coffee or tea!*

additional is going on in many people who have been using artificial sweeteners. The sweet taste of no-calorie sweeteners triggers an insulin release, even when there is no food intake to feed the cells.

Normally when we eat sugars, they are broken down into glucose, the form of sugar our body uses, which then enters the blood stream. Insulin, (secreted by the pancreas) unlocks the cells and allows blood sugar into our cells to supply energy and maintain normal blood sugar levels.

The problem is an insulin-sensitive person who uses artificial sweeteners confuses their body into thinking food has been eaten, so insulin is released. When insulin is released without food, it triggers the appetite.

As soon as your body discovers there is no food in your system, it creates strong cravings that can only be stopped by eating food that raises the blood sugar. It becomes pretty hard to avoid high-calorie sugary snacks at this point, and you get into a cycle of hunger, cravings and snacks.

Four artificial sweeteners have been approved by the FDA. In addition to saccharin (Sweet-n-Low®), sucralose (Splenda®) and aspartame (NutraSweet®, Equal®), there is acesulfame potassium, also called Ace-K and marketed as Sunette®, Sweet One® and Neotame®.

**Saccharin** was the first artificial sweetener on the market. Saccharin has no calories, and is hundreds of times sweeter than sugar. Many people notice an unpleasant, bitter aftertaste in foods sweetened with this product.

Saccharin has been a long-standing sugar substitute for many, with many faithful followers, but it has had issues related to health from the time it came out on the market. Saccharin is a synthetic, white crystalline powder. It has no nutritional value and is not easily digested by the body. It is still the third most popular artificial sweetener, after sucralose and aspartame.

Saccharin was discovered by accident in 1879. It was then commercialized, and almost immediately controversy started over its safety, which continues today.

In 1977, saccharin was accused of being a carcinogen after a study connected it to bladder tumors in mice. The U.S. National Toxicology Program then put saccharin on its cancer causing list—officially declaring it a human carcinogen. Cyclamate, an earlier version of the sweetener, had been banned in 1970 for similar reasons.

The American Food and Drug Administration decided it was prudent to mandate that saccharin carry a warning label regarding its cancer connection. The warning label has since been removed, due to inconclusive evidence of the saccharin and cancer connection in humans, but it is still a sweetener to be treated with caution, and certainly not healthy in the long run.

Saccharin (Sweet-n-Low®) can still cause these reactions in some sensitive people:

* Itching
* Hives
* Eczema
* Nausea
* Headaches
* Diarrhea
* Excessive urination
* Wheezing
* Tongue blisters

**Aspartame** has been on the market for over twenty years, and although there are many health concerns with the use of this artificial sweetener, it still remains a staple of the no-calorie artificial sweeteners, and is still commercially marketed in many products.

Aside from the weight gain problems, there are also large amounts of the population suffering from various unhealthy side effects associated with aspartame, although they may not even know it is the cause. Even individuals who do not have immediate reactions may still be susceptible to the long-term damage caused by the excitatory amino acids contained in aspartame: phenylalanine, methanol and DKP (aspartylphenylalanine diketopiperazine).

Adverse reactions and side effects of aspartame (NutraSweet®, Equal®) include:

* Vision problems
* Tinnitus - ringing or buzzing sounds
* Noise sensitivity or hearing impairment
* Epileptic seizures
* Headaches, migraines, dizziness
* Depression

* Irritability
* Aggression
* Anxiety, palpitations, tachycardia
* Stomach and abdominal pain
* Itching
* Rashes, hives

While **sucralose** seems to be safer than aspartame, there still has not been enough convincing evidence to prove its safety, and generally should be considered unsafe to use as a low-calorie sweetener.

Splenda®, the brand under which sucralose is marketed, claims to be "made from sugar," and "natural" because sucralose is a natural sugar.

According to Shane Ellison (www.thepeopleschemist.com), a well-known organic chemist:

*"Splenda®'s manufacturer claims that the chlorine added to sucralose is similar to the chlorine atom in the salt (NaCl) molecule. When combined with sodium, chlorine forms a harmless "ionic bond" to yield table salt. Sucralose makers often point this out to defend its safety. Apparently, they missed day two of Chemistry 101 - the day they taught about 'covalent' bonds. Unlike ionic bonds, covalently bound chlorines are not meant for the human body. Sucralose is covalently bonded with chlorine and much more like ingesting tiny amounts of chlorinated pesticides, but we will never know the real harm, without long- term, independent human research."*

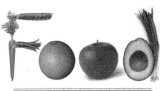

*for thought*

Sucralose is not at all natural; it is a chemically created synthetic compound, modified by adding chlorine atoms to sugar. It was discovered in the 1970s by researchers looking to create a new pesticide. It wasn't until the young scientist who developed it accidentally tasted his new "insecticide" that he learned it was sweet.

Since a no-calorie sweetener is much more marketable than a pesticide, it was named "Splenda®" and advertised as being a "natural" substitute for sugar. Little does the public know that this sweetener was once almost bug killer! If it kills bugs, it seems very likely that it is harmful to humans as well.

How does Splenda® work? Most of it passes through the body without being digested. Actually only around 10-15 percent of Splenda® is digested. People with healthier GI tracts end up absorbing more of the Splenda® because they are able to digest it, and that means more chlorine is absorbed into the body, along with the resulting health hazards.

Even tests done by Splenda®'s manufacturers are scary. Studies revealed that test animals suffered from some really nasty side effects such as enlarged livers and kidneys, and shrunken thymus glands…and these were only the short-term studies. What happens long-term?

Splenda® was rushed to the marketplace without any long-term studies done on it. It would seem that the long-term research is going on across America, with us as the test rodents.

If Splenda® is dangerous in smaller doses, what about larger amounts, along with the chlorine it contains? One of Splenda®'s selling points is that it remains stable at higher temperatures, meaning that it can be used in cooking, as opposed to the other low-calorie sweeteners.

The problem with that is many of the sugar-free and low-calorie diet foods now use Splenda® in their recipes. People on sugar-free and low-calorie diets are eating this product several times a day in different foods and drinks.

According to Dr. Joseph Mercola (www.mercola.com), the following symptoms have been observed within 24-hours of eating Splenda® products:

* Redness, itching, swelling, blistering, weeping, crusting, rash, eruptions, or hives. This is the most common allergic symptom that people have.
* Wheezing, tightness, cough, or shortness of breath.
* Swelling of the face, eyelids, lips, tongue, or throat; headaches and migraines.

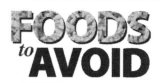

## SUGAR-FREE FOODS

*Diet sodas*

*Crystal Lite®*
*Lemonade Mixes*

*Sugar-Free Kool-Aid®*

*Sugar-free drinks*
*of all kinds*

*Sugar-free*
*sports drinks*

*Sugar-free snacks*
*and desserts*

*Sugar-free*
*ice-cream*

*Sugar-free syrups,*
*jams and jellies*

*Sugar-free gum*

*Sugar-free candy*

*Anything that says* **"Sugar free"** *read the label, most likely it contains one of the artificial sweeteners mentioned.*

* Stuffy nose, runny nose, sneezing.
* Red, itchy, swollen, or watery eyes.
* Bloating, gas, pain, nausea, vomiting,
    diarrhea, or bloody diarrhea.
* Heart palpitations or fluttering.
* Join pains or aches.
* Anxiety, dizziness, spaced-out
    sensation, depression.

Allergic reactions may not show up the first time, but may suddenly appear after several exposures. While it seems unlikely that sucralose is as toxic as aspartame, it is clear from the hazards seen in research, and from its chemical structure, that years and years of use may contribute to serious immunological and neurological disorders.

There are many other natural sweeteners that are much healthier choices and do not contain a list of frightening side effects when ingested.

New on the scene is a natural (non-artificial) sweetener derived from the stevia plant, called stevia. It is being marketed under several brand names such as Truvia® and Only Sweet®, to name two. This is an acceptable alternative as it is natural and does not cause a reaction from the pancreas to secrete insulin, nor does it alter blood sugar.

However, everything in moderation! It is best to alternate between natural sweeteners such as stevia, honey, maple syrup, molasses, organic agave nectar and xylitol (a sugar alcohol that doesn't effect the pancreas). Even natural sugar cane is acceptable in reserved amounts.

# 7 Good vs. Bad Fats

*Margarines, vegetable oils and trans fats*

We have all been told that we should avoid fat. The truth is, the right fats are a necessary part of a healthy diet, and they can actually make you leaner. Eating the wrong kinds of fat will not only make you fat, but contribute to a variety of other diseases and health issues as well as premature aging. Contrary to popular belief, unhealthy fats mostly include **trans fats** and **vegetable oils** - not cholesterol and saturated fats, as we have been led to believe.

Trans fats and vegetable oils are finally starting to get notice for being the villains of the health problems that they cause. It is these fats - not cholesterol and saturated fats - that are the primary contributors to inflammation, cancer, heart disease and obesity.

**Trans fats** are not natural fats. They are vegetable oils artificially created with hydrogen. This makes an oil turn into something more like a solid at room temperature. Food manufacturers use trans fats because they increase the shelf life of foods, but they are highly destructive in our bodies.

Eating trans fats is known to change your cell membranes and cause them to become brittle and unable to properly metabolize nutrients and calories. A healthy cell has a living, breathing membrane that transmits and utilizes nutrients properly. When you think of a cell affected by trans fats, think of a cell with a hard shell around it, instead of a healthy membrane. That shell actually smothers the cell, and causes the cell to become dysfunctional; blocking proper metabolism, nutrition, and creating an inability to respond to glucose. Inflammation in the body increases. This not only leads to diseases like diabetes and heart disease, but also weight gain, and an inability to fight infection and cancers.

Scientists have found that trans fat consumption decreased testosterone, caused the production of abnormal sperm, and altered gestation. Trans fat consumption also interferes with the body's use of the healthy omega-3 fatty acids found in fish oils, grains and green vegetables.

In spite of the dangers of trans fats, they are still found in many processed

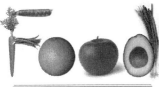

*for thought*

*Examples of vegetable oils are: canola oil, soybean oil, sunflower oil, corn oil, and safflower oil. Trans fat-containing foods include packaged cookies, crackers, desserts, margarine, and so-called "healthy" butter substitutes, Crisco®, buttered microwave popcorn, chips and more.*

and baked foods: cookies, crackers, cake icing, snack chips, stick margarine and microwave popcorn, to name just a few. Most of the trans fat in Americans' diets comes from commercially produced partially- or fully-hydrogenated vegetable oil. Margarine and any kind of substitute-butter spread, Crisco® and other solid shortenings are examples of trans fats. Butter is far better to eat than these artificial, unhealthy substitutes.

What about **vegetable oils**? Not so long ago, vegetable oil was thought to be a healthy alternative to saturated fat. Polyunsaturated vegetable oils were touted as the healthy oils to use over lard and animal fats. Keep in mind that the reason they were touted as "healthy" has to do with how cheap vegetable oils are to produce and the heavy marketing budgets behind the companies that push vegetable oils.

Oils like canola, corn, soybean and sunflower have been pushed as the healthy substitutes for more highly saturated fats. Sunflower oil and canola oils are still a popular choice for cooking. However, research has painted a very different picture. These oils contribute to inflammation in the body and upset the ratio of omega-3 fatty acids to omega-6 fatty acids.

Omega-3 fatty acids are the healthy fatty acids found in wild-caught fish and grass-fed meats. Omega-6 fatty acids are found in vegetable oils and trans fats. While omega-6 fatty acids are essential to our diet, they are consumed in amounts that are far too high for good health. Excess consumption of omega-6 oils leads to increased health problems, such as inflammatory-related diseases that include autoimmune diseases and cardiovascular disease.

The fats in our diet changed drastically in the early 1900s when refined vegetable oil, a major source of omega-6 fatty acids, entered the diet as margarine, and consumption of healthy, omega- 3 fatty acid foods, such as wild-caught fish, grass-fed beef, wild game and green, leafy vegetables, decreased. Our ancestors, the early hunter-gatherers, had a dietary omega-6 to omega-3 ratio of 2:1 or 3:1. This ratio today is about 20:1 in North America and most modernized diets around the world.

Consuming large amounts of vegetable oils is damaging to the body, especially the reproductive organs and the lungs, which have been sites for increases in cancer in the U.S. diets high in vegetable oils, especially hydrogenated vegetable oils, can cause irritability, learning disabilities, liver toxicity, decreased immune function, mental and physical growth problems in infants and children, increases in uric acid, abnormal fatty acid profiles in the fat tissue; and they have been linked to mental decline (Alzheimer's and dementia) and chromosomal damage because they accelerate aging.

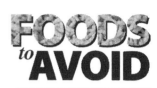

Excess consumption of vegetable oils and trans fats is associated with weight gain, cancer and heart disease. Vegetable oils, which are primarily omega-6 oils, are highly inflammatory; they interfere with the production of prostaglandins (inflammatory chemicals in the body) leading to a variety of health issues ranging from autoimmune diseases to PMS. This inflammation also leads to an increased tendency to form blood clots, which leads to heart attacks and strokes, now at epidemic levels in America.

Inflammation causes the arteries to send out cholesterol to repair the damage caused by the inflammation. When cholesterol is sent out by the body to repair damaged blood vessel walls, the cholesterol acts as a Band-Aid, covering the injury and building up on the vessel wall.

The cholesterol causes a buildup, and as the damage and inflammation continues the cholesterol begins to narrow the blood vessel, bringing on the beginning of atherosclerosis. Sad to say, cholesterol in the diet has been wrongly accused of being the culprit behind heart disease, but it is really the omega-6 fats as well as trans fats, sugars and other inflammatory foods in the average diet that are behind this health problem.

A 1994 study appearing in a leading medical journal showed that almost three quarters of the fat in clogged arteries is unsaturated. The "artery clogging"

## TRANS-FAT FOODS

*If you see ingredients that say anything related to "hydrogenated...oil,"* **AVOID** *them!*

*Margarine of any kind or any kind of butter substitute*
*Baked goods like cookies, doughnuts w/hydrogenated fats*
*Microwave popcorn*
*Crisco®*
*Frozen foods like french fries, TV dinners*
*Some peanut butters (natural peanut butters don't have added trans fats)*
*Cake icing*
*Frozen prepared meats like chicken tenders, etc.*
*Some whipped toppings*
*Cream substitutes*
*Fast food milk shakes*
*Velveeta® cheese or other processed packaged (squirt can) cheese*

fats are not animal fats, but vegetable oils! And way back in 1969, researchers discovered that the use of corn oil caused an increase in atherosclerosis.

Even the doctors and researchers who initially promoted the use of omega-6 vegetable oils as part of a healthy diet are now aware of their dangers. Scientists have actually warned against including too many polyunsaturated vegetable oils in the diet for several years.

Other research indicates that hydrogenated vegetable oils contribute to osteoporosis. And interestingly enough, a study done by a plastic surgeon found that people who consumed mostly vegetable oils had far more wrinkles than those who used traditional animal fats. So you see, these once so-called healthy oils are very aging to the body.

Vegetable oils are also more toxic when heated. One study reported that when these oils are heated, they turn to a varnish-like substance in the intestines. Have you ever tried to clean a pan with cooked-on vegetable oil? It's nearly impossible! Think of that happening inside your body! And heating vegetable oils over and over again increases the toxicity even more. Think of that the next time you get french fries. That oil has been heated to a high temperature many times!

Try this little trick next time you are thinking of ordering fries: Since we know that deep fryer oil is not only usually hydrogenated, but then also heated and reheated many times, and how all of this reacts almost as a poison inside your body, understanding this actually makes it easy to view deep-fried food like french fries as repulsive instead of something to crave.

There is absolutely **NOTHING** good about this poison! Avoid it all costs.

# 8 Commercial Pasteurized Dairy

*Although milk is typically promoted as a healthy food, there are many problems with commercial pasteurized dairy*

U nfortunately, virtually all of the milk sold in stores in the U.S. has been pasteurized (highly heated) and homogenized (treated so fat does not float to top), thus turning a healthy food into an unhealthy one. While the dairy industry is passing off pasteurized milk as being wholesome and healthy, it is far from that. Studies are showing evidence that commercial, pasteurized milk may play a role in a variety of health problems, including: diabetes, prostate cancer, rheumatoid arthritis, atherosclerosis, anemia, MS, leukemia and ovarian cancer.

There are dozens of reports and studies on pasteurized milk, and most of them are not favorable. Most of these published reports seem to be concerning the health issues that commercial, pasteurized milk causes such as: intestinal colic, intestinal irritation, intestinal bleeding, anemia, allergic and sinus problems, and salmonella. Contamination of milk by blood and white (pus) cells as well as a variety of hormones, chemicals and insecticides is also a big cause for concern.

### Bovine Growth Hormone

Did you know that fifty years ago, a cow produced 2,000 pounds of milk per year? Today the top producers produce close to 50,000 pounds! How can this be? It is certainly not a natural phenomenon. Drugs, antibiotics, forced feeding plans, specialized breeding and synthetic growth hormones are the causes.

The latest onslaught to the dairy cow is the addition of bovine growth hormone or rBGH. This is a synthetic hormone that is injected into cows to increase milk production. Developed and

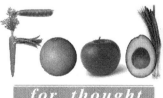

*for thought*

*There is only one form of healthy milk, and that is raw (unpasteurized, unhomogenized) milk from healthy, grass-fed cows.*

manufactured in the U.S. by the Monsanto Company, rBGH was approved by the FDA in 1993 despite opposition from scientists, farmers and consumers.

IGF-1, a naturally-occurring hormone found in the milk of both humans and cows that helps infants grow quickly, is stimulated by rBGH. In non-infants and adults, IGF-1 produces adverse effects and some researchers believe it acts as a cancer accelerator, with links to breast cancer (correlation shown in premenopausal women), prostate cancer, lung cancer and colon cancers.

Additionally, according to the European Union's Scientific Committee on Veterinary Measures Relating to Public Health, another factor to be considered is whether genetically-engineered hormone residues in milk and meat from "growth enhanced" animals can disrupt human hormone balance, cause developmental problems and interfere with the reproductive system. The group suggests that children, pregnant women and the unborn are the most susceptible to these negative health effects.

*For more information on the Monsanto Company and their work with genetically-modified corn, soybeans and cotton as well as agricultural herbicides and issues with allowing organic dairy farmers to label their milk "hormone free," go to http:// en.wikipedia.org/wiki/ Monsanto.*

Today's youth are reaching puberty at earlier and earlier ages. Hormone residues in beef have been implicated in the early onset of puberty in girls, which could put them at greater risk of developing breast and other forms of cancer, according to the European Commission. In addition, scientists have linked the rise in twin births over the last 30 years to bovine growth hormone in the food supply.

Many countries have banned rBGH because of safety concerns. And for good reason: Any substance added to a dairy cow's body comes out in the milk. All mammals who are lactating excrete many toxins through their milk, and this includes antibiotics, pesticides, chemicals and growth hormones.

According to The Monsanto Company, rBGH does not affect the milk or meat of injected cattle. Can such claims be believed? Amidst continued controversy and lawsuits over this issue, Monsanto sold its POSILAC Bovine Somatropin brand and related bovine growth hormone business to Elanco Animal Health, a division of Eli Lilly and Company, in August, 2008.

Obviously, there have been no long-term studies on the hormone's effect on humans drinking milk containing rBGH, but some studies have focused on rBGH and the growth of cancerous tumors. It makes perfect sense that if this unnatural drug can stimulate growth, then it can stimulate the growth of cancer, hormones and other cells within a body as well.

## *Antibiotics*

Because rBGH dramatically increases the cow's milk supply, it also causes a dramatic increase (50 to 70 percent) in mastitis (udder infections) in the dairy cows' udders. This in turn then requires antibiotics to get rid of the mastitis, and the leftover antibiotics then appear in the milk we drink.

Over 50 percent of all the antibiotics produced in this country for both humans and animals go directly into animal feed! Ideally, antibiotics should be used in farming only when necessary to treat infections. But commercial dairy cows are raised in poor, dirty conditions, and they are not healthy animals. So they are fed a constant supply of antibiotics from birth until death.

We are unknowingly consuming a lot of antibiotics, just by drinking commercial milk. Because of this, humans are now becoming resistant to antibiotics. If you tested commercial milk, you would find that it contains traces of up to 80 different antibiotics!

Because of the mastitis, there are white blood cells – also referred to as pus - in the milk from infections. Inspectors are asked to keep the white blood cell counts under certain limits. A not-too-appetizing fact is that the USDA allows milk to contain from one to one-and-a-half million white blood cells per milliliter. That's one to one-and-a- half million WBCs to about 1/30 of an ounce.

Pure, wholesome milk? Yuck! It is now a disgusting cocktail of antibiotics, chemicals, hormones and pus. Do you want yourself – or you children – to be the guinea pigs for such an experiment?

## *Pasteurization*

But wait, there's more! Pasteurization further degrades milk and makes it even more unhealthy. As we mentioned earlier, commercially raised dairy cattle are raised under dirty, unhealthy conditions. In addition, most commercial dairy cows are raised on an unnatural diet of grains, not grass like Mother Nature intended. Because this diet is so unnatural for the cows, this totally changes the composition of the fats in milk, primarily the very important and healthy fatty acids: Omega 3s and conjugated linoleic acid.

Raw milk sours naturally, but pasteurized milk will turn putrid, and processors remove slime and pus from pasteurized milk by a process of centrifugal clarification.

What's more, inspection of commercial dairy cows for disease is not even required for pasteurized milk. So, dirty, crowded, dairy lots are full of sickly cattle that are giving us milk!

Pasteurizing milk actually began in the 1920s to kill pathogens that got into the milk that caused Tuberculosis, infant diarrhea, intestinal dysentery, and other diseases brought on by poor animal nutrition and dirty production methods. According to Sally Fallon of the Weston Price Foundation, a U.S. non-profit dedicated to restoring nutrient-dense foods to the American diet through education, research and activism:

*"Heat alters milk's amino acids, lysine and tyrosine, making the whole complex of proteins less available; it promotes rancidity of unsaturated fatty acids and destruction of vitamins. Vitamin C loss in pasteurization usually exceeds 50 percent; loss of other water-soluble vitamins can run as high as 80 percent. Pasteurization alters milk's mineral components such as calcium, chlorine, magnesium, phosphorus, potassium, sodium and sulphur as well as many trace minerals, making them less available. There is some evidence that pasteurization alters lactose, making it more readily absorbable."*

When milk is pasteurized, the protein molecules are heated and they actually change shape and composition, making them much harder for our bodies to break down and digest. A simple protein molecule becomes a tightly folded molecule. This milk then puts an unnecessary strain on our digestive system to produce digestive enzymes to break this down. Many people's bodies are simply incapable of breaking this protein down.

This is partly the reason why milk consumption has been linked with diabetes. It is a strain on the pancreas to produce enzymes. It is also the reason behind many milk allergies. It is the protein portion— the casein--that becomes difficult to digest after pasteurization, thus causing many reactions.

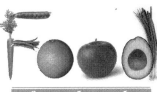

*Commercial pasteurized milk is not a health food and should be avoided at all costs. It is just empty calories that add pounds to your body, and fill you with chemicals.*

In the elderly, and those with milk intolerance or other digestive disorders, the milk passes through the intestinal walls not fully digested. These large particles can clog the absorbent areas of the small intestine, which then prevents vital nutrients from getting in. The result is allergies, chronic fatigue, lowered immune system and a variety of other degenerative diseases.

Because the milk is heated in pasteurization, the heat destroys the active and healthy enzymes in milk–in fact, the test for successful pasteurization is absence of enzymes. These enzymes are especially important to help our body break down and use all the healthy nutrients in milk, including calcium. This is why people with osteoporosis cannot get calcium from pasteurized milk. The calcium in milk is simply not utilized very well.

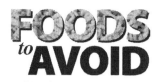

**COW'S MILK
PRODUCTS**

*Pasteurized cow's
    milk, even organic
    cow's milk
Pasteurized cottage
    cheese
Pasteurized yogurt
Pasteurized sour
    cream
Pasteurized,
    processed cheese
Pasteurized
    chocolate milk
Pasteurized cream
Any pasteurized
    processed dairy
    product*

The same goes for the healthy fats milk contains. Lipase is one of the enzymes in raw milk that helps the body digest and utilize the butterfat that contains conjugated linoleic acid (CLA) and omega-3 fats— both extremely healthy to the body in their cancer-fighting and heart- healthy abilities as well as helping with fat burning and muscle building.

Last but not least, there may be chemicals after pasteurization to suppress any rotten milk odor and restore some of the taste. Synthetic vitamin D2 or D3 is added – D2 is toxic and has been linked to heart disease while D3 is difficult to absorb.

Because it is cosmetically better looking, milk is then homogenized. Homogenization has lately been linked to heart disease and atherosclerosis. When you get milk straight from the cow it contains cream, which is full of all the healthy fats, including the fat-burning CLA. Homogenization breaks up the fat particles into smaller, microscopic particles and distributes the fat throughout the milk so that they do not rise. This process unnaturally increases the surface area of fat exposing it to air. Oxidation occurs and increases the susceptibility to spoilage.

Considering how commercial milk is produced and processed, it comes as no surprise that so many of us are allergic to it.

An allergic reaction to dairy can cause symptoms like:

* Diarrhea
* Vomiting (even projectile vomiting)
* Stomach pain
* Depression
* Cramping
* Gas
* Bloating
* Nausea

* Headaches
* Sinus and chest congestion
* Acne
* A sore or scratchy throat

Commercial milk consumption has been linked to many other health conditions as well, such as asthma, atherosclerosis, diabetes, chronic infections (especially upper respiratory and ear infections), obesity, osteoporosis and cancer of the prostate, ovaries, breast and colon.

Once you understand how modern milk is produced and processed, it seems logical to just avoid pasteurized, processed milk altogether. Why add the empty calories, antibiotics and growth hormones? Raw, unpasteurized, unhomogenized milk from healthy grass-fed cows is the best source of milk to drink. See more about raw milk in Part 2 of this manual.

If you must consume milk and milk products, do it in small quantities and make sure it is low fat and organic.

# 9

# Commercially Raised Meats and Farmed Fish

*Not all meat and fish are the same*

C ommercial production has sadly changed meat and fish from healthy, lean proteins into industrialized factory food with fewer nutrients that is now a health hazard. The animals raised for commercial meat sold in most grocery stores are bred and raised in captivity, fed an unhealthy diet that is not the natural diet of the animal, and slaughtered in inhumane, cruel conditions. This results in an unhealthy meat product for your consumption. But read on because there ARE healthy meats from which you can choose.

## *Grain-fed vs. Grass-fed Beef*

Most beef cattle start out on a range, eating grass, but upon reaching maturity, they are transported to a feedlot to be fattened and readied for slaughter. They spend their last few months at feedlots, crowded by the thousands into dusty, manure-laden holding pens. The air is thick with harmful bacteria, infectious disease, and dusty matter, putting the cattle at risk for respiratory disease and other diseases. Eventually, all of them will wind up at the slaughterhouse.

Feedlot cattle are injected regularly with growth hormones and antibiotics. Because they are fed an unnatural diet of grain and other food by-products - to fatten them up very quickly for profit - the cattle often have upset digestive systems, and they become even sicker and unhealthier in general.

Grains (often contaminated with fungus and fungicides) are used to fatten up livestock at the expense of their natural diet of healthy grass and hay. The main ingredients are genetically modified grain and soy. To further cut costs, the feed may also contain "by-product feedstuff" such as municipal garbage, stale pastry, chicken feathers, gum and candy.

Because cattle are naturally suited to eating a grass-based diet, the high-calorie diet of grain contributes to many metabolic disorders. Cattle fed a grain-based diet also develop highly acidic stomachs to process the grain. This acidic environment is the breeding ground for the deadly E-coli strain of bacteria that sickens and kills many people.

In the U.S. alone, farmers add 10 million pounds of antibiotics into the food and water supply of farm animals. This, however, is not intended to fight

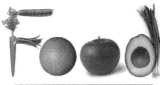

*for thought*

*Since the 1980s, mergers and acquisitions have resulted in concentrating 80 percent of the 35 million beef cattle slaughtered annually in the U.S. into the hands of four huge corporations. What used to be idyllic country farms with contented grazing cattle has turned into huge, industrialized factory farms with unhealthy feedlots.*

or prevent disease, but is actually used to fatten up the livestock, which is one of the side effects of the antibiotics. All of the antibiotics in the meat you are eating – as well as in the milk, as mentioned earlier - can lead to antibiotic resistance in your body. And, if these antibiotics work to fatten cattle, it's not out of the question to think they may be contributing to fattening humans!

Cattle are transported several times during their lifetimes, and they can travel hundreds or thousands of miles during a single trip. Long journeys are very stressful to the cattle, and contribute to even more disease and death.

A standard beef slaughterhouse kills about 250 cattle an hour. The high speed of the processing makes it difficult to treat animals humanely. According to a meat industry article, "Good handling is extremely difficult if equipment is 'maxed out' all the time. It is impossible to have a good attitude towards the cattle if the employees are stressed and constantly rushed, trying to up their production in as little time as possible."

All that stress gets transferred to the animals, which is partly accountable for some of the terribly inhumane treatment cattle get.

Nearly all the meat, eggs and dairy products that you find in the supermarket come from animals raised in large facilities called CAFOs or "Confined Animal Feeding Operations." These highly mechanized operations provide a year-round supply of food at a reasonable price. Although the meat is cheap and convenient, factory farming is creating a variety of problems, including:

* Animal sickness, stress and abuse
* Air, land and water pollution
* The unnecessary use of hormones, antibiotics and other drugs that end
      up in the meat you are eating
* Unhealthy fats that cause inflammation and heart disease
* Food with decreased nutritional value

As detailed in Chapter 7: Good vs. Bad Fats, saturated fat is not the real culprit in heart disease and other degenerative diseases. It is the large amounts of inflammatory (hence, artery clogging) omega-6 fatty acids.

The fat in a grain-fed cow is not healthy, as it contains high amounts of omega-6 fatty acids.

One reason Americans are so unhealthy and have a lot of inflammation in their bodies is due to excessively high amounts of processed omega-6 fatty acids in our diets compared to far too low amounts of omega-3 fatty acids.

According to the Journal of Animal Science, grain-fed beef or bison can have an omega 6 to omega 3 ratio higher than 20:1, which we learned earlier is far beyond the healthy recommended ratio of 2:1 or 3:1. On the other hand, grass-fed beef or bison typically contain a much healthier omega-6 to omega-3 ratio of between 2:1 to 4:1 as well as much higher quantities of CLA.

Animals raised on their natural diet of grass have a healthy, highly functioning pH of 7, which allows for the essential fermentation of bacteria in their stomachs that creates high levels of nutrients, such as: CLA, omega-3 fats, branch-chain amino acids, vitamins, minerals and digestive enzymes. But even a small amount of grain can throw all this off. Just 30 days on a grain-based diet can ruin 200 days of grass-grazing chemistry.

When an animal lives on a high starch grain diet, the healthy pH 7 suddenly drops to a highly acidic pH 4. With this increase in acidity comes a different problem, one that stops the production of healthy fats like omega-3s and CLA, and increases the level of the omega-6s, of which most Americans already consume too much.

And as if all that weren't bad enough, the growth hormones that are given to fatten the cattle for faster weight gain don't create healthy, lean muscle. With less exercise than their pasture-raised, grass fed counterparts, grain-fed cattle develop heavy, highly marbled muscle mass that is the hallmark of their high-carbohydrate, high starch diet. Interesting thought...could this be happening in our bodies on a high carbohydrate, starchy diet as well?

When animals are raised in feedlots or cages, they leave behind large amounts of manure in a small amount of space. Manure must be collected and transported away from the area, which becomes an expensive proposition. It is usually dumped as close to the feedlot as possible to help defray the cost of removing it. As a result, the surrounding soil is overloaded with not only manure, but the residue of hormones and antibiotics from the cattle, which can cause ground and water pollution.

### *Farmed fish vs. Wild-caught fish*

Just as the commercial meat industry in America has now industrialized factory farms, producing thousands of pounds of unhealthy meats to meet consumer demand, now there's a similar dynamic in the global fish farming, or aquaculture, industry - especially as it strains to satisfy consumers' voracious appetite for top-of-the-food chain, carnivorous fish, such as salmon and tuna.

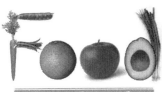

*Choose smaller fish such as sardines, herring, sunfish, trout and salmon and avoid large fish such as tuna, swordfish, shark, striped bass and blue fish.*

While fish used to be considered a healthy addition to any diet, farmed fish is now no better than eating a Big Mac®. From both a nutritional and environmental impact perspective, farmed fish are far inferior to their wild counterparts:

Despite being much fattier, farmed fish provide less usable beneficial omega 3 fats than wild fish.

Due to the feedlot conditions of aqua farming, farm-raised fish are doused with antibiotics and exposed to more concentrated pesticides than their wild kin.

Farmed salmon are given a salmon-colored dye in their feed, without which their flesh would be an unappetizing grey color.

Aqua farming also raises a number of environmental concerns, the most important of which may be its negative impact on wild salmon. It has now been established that sea lice from farms kill up to 95 percent of juvenile wild salmon that migrate past them.

There are numerous nutritional differences between farm-raised and wild fish.

Farm-raised fish have a higher fat content. It's not very surprising, since farm-raised fish do not spend their lives vigorously swimming through cold ocean waters or leaping up rocky streams like their wild counterparts. A marine version of couch potatoes, they circle lazily in crowded pens, fattening up on pellets of grain-based fish chow.

In each of the species evaluated by the USDA, the farm-raised fish were found to contain more total fat than their wild counterparts. For rainbow trout, the difference in total fat was the smallest, while cultivated catfish had nearly five times as much fat as wild catfish. Farm-raised Coho salmon had approximately three times the total fat as wild samples.

Farm-raised fish contain more inflammatory omega-6 fats, and an imbalance of omega-6 to omega-3 fatty acids. In three types of fish evaluated, the amount of omega-6 fats was substantially higher in farm-raised compared to wild fish. The total of all types of omega-6 fats found in cultivated fish was at least twice the level found in the wild samples.

Generally, you can figure that farm-raised fish will have 10-30 percent more fat (and that's mostly omega-6 fats, which you already get too much of) and calories than wild-caught fish.

The fat in farmed salmon contains far less of the healthy omega-3 fatty acids than the fat in wild salmon. Salmon fat is usually rich in omega-3 fatty acids. Not so with farmed fish!

Disease and parasites, which would normally exist in relatively low levels in fish scattered around the oceans, can run rampant in densely-packed oceanic feedlots. To survive, farmed fish are vaccinated as minnows. Later, they are given antibiotics or pesticides to ward off infection.

Sea lice, in particular, are one of the worst problems. While salmon farmers have discounted concerns that sea lice are also found in the wild, at the first sign of an outbreak, they add pesticides to the feed.

Scientists in the United States are far more concerned about two studies, both of which showed farmed salmon accumulate more cancer-causing PCBs (polychlorinated biphenyl) and poisonous dioxins than wild salmon. PCBs and similarly-classed dioxins are classified as a "persistent organic pollutants," and were banned from production in the United States in 1979. Toxic effects such as endocrine disruption and nuerotoxicity are associated with these compounds.

*Note : When you're choosing healthier wild fish, it is a good idea to try to limit your intake of fish that are higher on the food chain (such as tuna, swordfish, shark, striped bass, bluefish, etc.) to more occasional meals due to the higher levels of mercury in these fish.*

Tests on farmed salmon sold at grocery stores - which contains up to twice the fat of wild salmon - has found 16 times the PCBs compared to wild salmon, 4 times the levels in commercial beef, and 3.5 times the levels found in other seafood. Most of these toxins are stored in the fat of the fish, so guess what you are eating when you eat farmed fish?

Farmed salmon usually has dye added to it to improve the looks of the product. Even with the coloring, it never looks as good as wild salmon. These colorings also come with recently documented cancer-causing agents. These dyes have zero health benefits, and have no other purpose than to fool you, the consumer, into thinking the product is rich in flavor. Don't believe it!

Aqua farms, or "floating pig farms," put a major strain on the surrounding environment. The fish consume huge amounts of highly-concentrated protein pellets

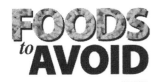

## MEATS/FISH PRODUCTS

*Packaged, commercially sold grocery store beef of all cuts*

*Packaged, processed meats like bacon, salami, bologna, hot dogs, sausage, etc (high levels of sodium, nitrates or nitrites, and preservatives).*

*Frozen prepared meats*

*Canned meats, processed chipped beef*

*Any kind of fish that says "farm-raised"*

*Processed or fried fish such as fish sticks, etc.*

*Frozen diet dinners*

*Fast food burgers, fast food fish*

and it makes a terrific mess.

Uneaten feed and fish waste cover the ocean floor beneath these farms, which are a breeding ground for bacteria that consume oxygen vital to shellfish and other bottom-dwelling sea creatures. A good-sized salmon farm produces an amount of excrement equivalent to the sewage of a city of 10,000 people. Think about that the next time you swim in the ocean!

The most serious concern is the depletion of marine life from over-fishing. Actually, aqua farming depletes marine life because captive salmon are carnivores and must be fed fish during the two to three year period when they are raised. To produce one pound of farmed salmon, two to four pounds of wild sardines, anchovies, mackerel, herring and other fish must be ground up to render the oil and meal that is compressed into pellets of salmon chow.

Fish used to be a bit of a rarity in U.S. households. Today it is a common dinner at the homes of health-conscious consumers. Last year, salmon overtook "fish sticks" as the third most popular seafood in the American diet (trailing tuna and shrimp). The increased consumption was made possible by the explosive growth in salmon farming, an industrial system that produces the fish in vast quantities at a price far lower than wild salmon.

Another popular fish for consumers is Tilapia. Although portrayed as "healthy," most tilapia sold at restaurants and grocery stores is farm raised, and therefore is not considered the healthiest of choices.

More than half of the fish sold in supermarkets, fish markets and restaurants are raised in high-density fish pens in the ocean, managed and marketed by the farmed fishing industry. These fish are eaten by over a quarter of all adults in the U.S. and experts predict that the exponential growth of the farmed fish industry will continue. Although it seems like a healthier choice, eating farmed fish is actually almost as bad as eating a fast food burger.

Fish that are lower on the food chain, such as sardines, herring, sunfish, and even trout and salmon, have lower levels of mercury and are not as much of a concern.

*Caution: it is extremely important for pregnant women to speak to your doctor about fish intake.*

# 10 All About Soy

*Including genetically modified soy
(GMO) and isolated soy protein*

S oy as health food? Think again! Only a few decades ago, the soybean (unfermented) was considered unfit to eat - even in Asia. Here, it is touted as a food superstar.

The soybean was not considered as food until the discovery of fermentation techniques around 1027A.D. to 221 B.C. Soy as food was always in fermented form like tempeh, natto, miso and soy sauce.

Unfermented soy contains growth-suppressing agents. When the growth-blocking agents were lowered by fermenting, soy began as a dietary staple. But the soybean was always fermented first, never eaten in its unfermented form.

Unfermented soybeans were never eaten because soybeans contain large quantities of natural toxins which are actually "anti-nutrients." These anti-nutrients block enzymes that are necessary for digestion and assimilation.

The natural toxins in soy can produce serious gastric distress and difficulties in digesting proteins and amino acids.

Some of these natural toxins in soybeans are growth inhibitors, and since they block nutrient absorption, they should never be fed to children and babies.

Soybeans and other legumes contain large amounts of a substance called phytic acid. Phytic acid can be found in hulls of beans or seeds. It will block essential minerals - calcium, magnesium, copper, iron and especially zinc - in the intestinal tract from being absorbed.

Soybeans typically contain one of the highest phytate levels of any legume, and long, slow heating or cooking will not help to reduce this substance. Only fermenting techniques will lower this nutrient blocker.

Phytate content can also be reduced by eating meat with the soy. In many oriental dishes, soy is often consumed in a meal that has meat as a part of the menu.

So then, if you are a vegetarian, eating tofu and soy products as a substitute for meat and protein, it will cause nutritional deficiencies. Not only does the risk of B12 deficiency go way up, but mineral deficiencies are common as well. Zinc, calcium, magnesium and iron deficiencies have all been noted, but zinc deficiency is often the worst. Sometimes these deficiencies may show up as unnatural cravings for foods like chocolate and other less- than-healthy foods.

Zinc is necessary for a strong immune system and also plays a role in intelligence and behavior because it is needed for optimal development and functioning of the brain and nervous system. Zinc is very important to protein synthesis and collagen formation; it is involved in blood-sugar control, helps protect against diabetes, and it is needed for a healthy reproductive system.

While soy food companies strive to remove these nutrient-blocking substances from the finished product, soy protein isolate (SPI) is the primary protein component in most soy foods that imitate meat and dairy products, and also baby formulas and some brands of soy milk.

What is soy protein isolate? Well, don't be fooled, it is not a naturally occurring substance. Soybeans are made into a slurry and combined with an alkaline solution to remove fiber, and then separated using an acid wash and, finally, neutralized in an alkaline solution. Does this sound like something you want to eat?

When this soy mixture is acid washed, it is usually done in aluminum tanks, which then leach aluminum into the soy products. Soy curds are spray-dried at high temperatures to produce a protein powder. This high temperature, high-pressure process then creates TVP or textured vegetable (or soy) protein. The high temperature processing actually denatures the protein, making it virtually useless.

Nitrites (a potent cancer-causing agent) are created in the spray drying process, and a toxin called lysinoalanine is formed during alkaline processing. Does soy still sound like the healthy super food you thought it was?

Experiments using soy protein isolate created deficiencies of vitamins E, D, B12, calcium, magnesium, manganese, molybdenum, copper, iron and zinc. The test animals also developed enlarged organs such as the pancreas and thyroid gland, and fatty livers.

You don't have to be a vegetarian to be eating soy protein isolate and textured vegetable protein. They are heavily used in school lunch programs, commercial baked goods, diet foods and fast food products as well as meat substitutes and energy bars. They are heavily promoted in third world countries and are a main part of many food giveaway programs to starving people.

Advances in technology make it possible to produce isolated soy protein from what used to be a waste product - defatted, high-protein soy chips - and then transformed from something that looks and smells ghastly into products that will be consumed by human beings. Added flavorings, preservatives, sweeteners, emulsifiers and synthetic nutrients change soy protein isolate into a seemingly delicious manufactured food.

Soy is now marketed to the health-conscious, upscale consumer as a miracle substance that will prevent heart disease and cancer, whisk away hot flashes, build strong bones and keep us healthy and slender.

In the process of creating the image in everyone's mind of soy as a healthy super food, meat, milk, cheese, butter and eggs have become the bad guys in the food pyramid instead of being portrayed as the wholesome healthy foods they truly are. Soy has replaced meat and dairy products for vegetarians and health-conscious consumers, and gets marketed as being a "healthy" replacement for meat, fish and eggs to escape the so-called evils of saturated fat and cholesterol. In reality, it's much worse.

Soy's positive effects on cholesterol levels are questionable, say scientists. In addition, studies in which cholesterol levels were lowered through either diet or drugs have actually resulted in a greater number of deaths in the treatment groups than in controls - deaths from stroke, cancer, intestinal disorders, accident and suicide.

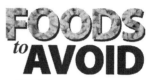

Soy contains plant estrogens that, although touted by soy advocates as healthy and good for women, are phytoestrogens that can actually disrupt hormones in the body and cause potential harm. And if you are a man, should you be ingesting soy loaded with substances that mimic female hormones? High soy consumption can actually contribute to male breast growth (a.k.a, "man boobs" - gynecomastia)!

Soy disrupts the digestive, immune and neuro-endocrine systems of the human body and plays a major role in infertility, hypothyroidism and some types of cancer, including thyroid and pancreatic cancers. Does this sound like health food?

Soy is one of the top ten food allergens, and some rate it fifth or sixth highest of allergenic foods. Allergic reactions to soy are increasingly common, ranging from mild to life threatening. A little-known fact about some food allergies: they create a craving for the very food you are allergic to, turning into a vicious cycle of craving and eating and more reactions, which leads to more weight gain.

It should be obvious that soy is not a miracle food, and it certainly is not a health food!

### SOY FOODS
*Soy milk*
*Soy baby formula*
*Powdered soy protein*
*Tofu*
*Frozen soy "ice cream" products like Tofutti Cuties®*
*Soy protein energy bars (look at the ingredients as soy protein hides in MOST so-called "energy" bars/protein bars)*
*Textured vegetable protein as an ingredient in meatless products or as a thickener*
*Tofurky*
*Tofu hot dogs*
*MorningStar® products*
*Soy snacks, soy chips, soy and rice cake snacks*
*Meatless burgers*
*Meatless fast food meals*

# 11 Sports and Energy Drinks

*Helping performance or adding empty calories?*

A thletes everywhere pick up sports drinks to quench their thirst and replenish carbohydrates. Do they really work? Do energy and sports drinks help performance or do they just add empty calories?

Slick and entertaining advertising campaigns and celebrity athlete spokespersons give many people the impression that these drinks are healthy and essential during or after a workout to replace lost electrolytes, carbohydrates and fluids.

Although simple carbohydrates are helpful for athletes engaging in high-intensity exercise, are sports drinks effective, or even appropriate, for the average gym member or weekend warrior?

In one study, researchers prepared beverages containing glucose, maltodextrin or neither so that they tasted identical, and gave them to athletes, who rinsed the drinks around in their mouths before spitting them out during exercise. Despite not reaping the energizing effects of the carbohydrates in the drinks, the rinsing of the simple sugar mixes were shown to "significantly reduce the time to complete the cycle time trial," while the placebo drinks had no such effect. Researchers concluded that most of the benefit from carbohydrates in sports drinks is provided by signaling directly from mouth to brain rather than providing energy for the working muscle.

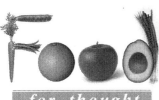
*for thought*

*Sports drinks can be up to 30 times more erosive to your teeth than water.*

Another study found that citric acid, commonly found in sports drinks, ate away at the enamel coating on teeth. As a result, the drinks could easily leak into the bone-like material underneath, causing a weakening and softening of the tooth that could result in severe tooth damage and even tooth loss if left untreated.

A recent study pointed out that brushing your teeth will not help because the citric acid in the sports drink will soften tooth enamel so much it could be damaged just by brushing.

According to researchers at the University of New Mexico, "Unless a person is going to exercise for at least 90 minutes, consuming the carbohydrates is self-defeating."

While sports drinks containing carbohydrates may help the body absorb water, there's no evidence that your body will retain water more effectively than if you just drank water alone, so they are really not more effective at battling dehydration.

The leading brands of sports drinks on the market typically contain as much as two-thirds the sugar of sodas and more sodium. They also often contain high-fructose corn syrup (HFCS), artificial flavors and food coloring - none of which belong in your body, and none of which are healthy.

If you are exercising to lose weight and get into shape, you should know that sports drinks and energy drinks will cause weight gain, similar to drinking soda. It is a sad irony that many people work hard and sweat to lose weight, only to gain weight from drinking sports drinks.

And although these drinks are often referred to as "energy" drinks, in the long run the sugar they contain does just the opposite. A quick explosion of energy is followed by a plummet in blood sugar, as your system floods with insulin to balance out your blood sugar. So the quick energy you may feel from the sugar soon becomes less energy as your blood sugar drops. And lo and behold, hunger cravings start as soon as the blood sugar drops.

Because it is metabolized by the liver, the fructose in high fructose corn syrup (which is the common sweetener in most sports drinks) does not cause the pancreas to release insulin the way it normally does. Fructose converts to fat more quickly than any other sugar. Fructose raises triglycerides significantly.

For complete conversion of fructose into glucose your body needs it must rob ATP energy stores from the liver. ATP is the fuel which supplies the energy to muscles, especially while exercising. If you are robbing your muscles' energy stores, then your sports drink is actually decreasing your athletic performance! So now you are tired and weaker from drinking sports drinks.

If your sports drink is low calorie and sugar-free, then it most likely contains an artificial sweetener, which is even worse for you than high-fructose corn syrup or sugar. And don't think that because a sports drink claims to be low-or no-calorie that it won't contribute to weight gain. As mentioned before, artificial sweeteners are as big a culprit in weight gain as sugar and corn syrup.

Sports drinks also contain large quantities of salt, which is there to replace electrolytes. But, unless you're sweating profusely and for a prolonged period, that extra salt is simply unnecessary, and possibly harmful. Too much of concentrated electrolytes can actually throw off your body's delicate electrolyte balance as well.

The excess salt will actually make you thirstier and make you want to drink more, while causing you to retain water and feel heavier and look bloated. You may think you are doing your body good, but drinking sports drinks are no better than drinking soda after your workout.

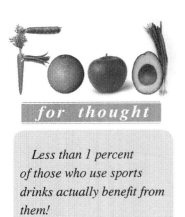

*Less than 1 percent of those who use sports drinks actually benefit from them!*

Unless you are exercising for more than 60 minutes at a time, sports drinks are unnecessary. It's only when you've been exercising for longer periods, such as 60 minutes or more, or at an extreme intensity, such as on a very hot day or at your full exertion level, that you may need something more than water to replenish your body.

Anything less than 45 minutes will not result in a large enough fluid loss to justify using these high-sodium, high-sugar drinks. Stay slim and lean and drink water!

Energy drinks were popularized in the U.S. with the introduction of Red Bull®, a carbonated beverage from Austria that contains 80 mg of caffeine in every bottle —about the same amount as is found in a cup of coffee. For comparison, classic Coca Cola® contains 23 mg of caffeine and Mountain Dew® contains 37 mg of caffeine.

Other brands of energy drinks may contain twice as much or more caffeine as Red Bull ®, plus other questionable ingredients such as guarana — a South American caffeine-containing herb.

The calories in these drinks do provide some energy, but mostly their content of caffeine, guarana and taurine turn up one's feelings of alertness and may produce troublesome side effects such as anxiety, irritability, heart palpitations, difficulty sleeping, and indigestion.

These occurrences are more likely to happen with energy drinks than with coffee, which is usually drunk more slowly than chilled energy drinks. Energy drinks can also lead to dehydration because the caffeine stimulates urination and thus increases water and electrolyte loss. Dehydration during athletic activities not only drastically reduces performance, but also can cause painful muscle cramping.

# 12 Energy and Protein Bars

*Candy bars in disguise*

They claim to be healthy, while looking and tasting like candy bars, but contain protein and fiber and are advertised as containing vitamins and minerals. Energy and protein bars are convenient and they taste good.

We'll share with you at the end of this section a few rare, healthy energy bars, but most are just candy bars in disguise.

The original energy bars, like the Power Bar® and the Source Bar®, were based on so-called "natural" sweeteners—high fructose corn syrup and juice concentrates—along with dried fruits and nuts. This combination resulted in higher percentages of carbohydrates than the typical chocolate candy bar, which is rich in cocoa butter, a healthy natural fat.

When cheap soy and whey proteins became available, the energy bar industry exploded, now that protein could be added to make a "high-protein" bar. Balance Bars® ("The Complete Nutritional Food Bar"), ZonePerfect Bars® ("All Natural Nutrition Bars"), and Atkins Bars® were among the first to hit the shelves as energy/protein bars.

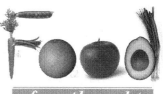

*Somehow we have been duped into thinking energy/protein bars are healthy snack food, or worse yet, a meal replacement.*

Sadly, there is nothing natural about the protein used in today's energy bars. Most bars are made with highly-processed soy protein (see the chapter on soy products). Isolated soy protein comes with an initial burden of nutrient-blocking agents such as phytic acid, enzyme inhibitors and isoflavones. Soy protein is processed at very high temperatures to reduce the levels of phytic acid and enzyme inhibitors; a process that degrades many of the proteins in soy, making them useless as usable protein in the body. Much of the soy in energy bars is genetically modified as well. More toxins are formed during high-temperature, high-pressure chemical processing, including nitrates, lysinalanine and MSG.

The other protein frequently used in energy bars is whey protein, which must be processed at low temperatures or the protein will be destroyed. When cheese, butter and cream were produced on farms in the past, the whey and skim milk used to be given to the pigs and chickens. Now that cheese, butter and cream are processed in industrial food factories far from farms, the dairy industry has an overabundance of whey.

The problem of what to do with this byproduct is solved by drying the skim milk and whey at high temperatures and putting the powders into energy drinks, bodybuilding powders and high-protein bars. But the protein content in most processed whey is damaged by the heat, so it is not the protein source it claims to be.

One major ingredient in energy bars is high-fructose corn syrup, an ingredient that has been shown to be worse than sugar and in humans causes insulin levels to spike as that sugar overloads our systems. Other major ingredients such as fiber from oats, apples, soy and citrus provide fiber. Sometimes maltodextrin is given as the fiber source. "Natural flavors" and piles of synthetic vitamins are thrown in so the bars can be called "complete."

On the good side, the fat source in most energy bars is often palm, palm kernel, or coconut oil, and so they are somewhat better than hydrogenated oils and trans fats, which are far worse for you.

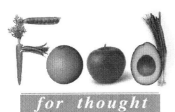

*Some good alternatives to energy bars for quick healthy snacks on the go could be as simple as a bag of mixed raw nuts (almonds, pecans, walnuts, etc.) with a little bit of dried fruit (just be careful not to eat large amounts of dried fruit due to the high sugar content).*

With the exception of the fats, most of the ingredients used in energy bars are industrial food waste products. Soy protein isolate and whey protein are the waste products of the soy oil and dairy industries. Apple and lemon fiber, often used to create a crunchy effect, are also waste, made from the pulp left over from squeezing the fruits for their juice. Soy lecithin, another common ingredient, is also a waste product of the soy oil industry. And, most of the sweeteners are made by highly industrialized processes. So you see, the ingredients in most energy and protein bars are anything but natural!

While many of the modern energy bars emphasize athletic performance, others are said to promote optimal mental performance. The Think! Nutrition Bar® claims that it will bestow "concentration, calmness, stamina. For best

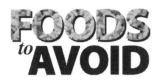

results," says the label, "eat a Think! Nutrition® bar and 16 ounces of fresh water 30 minutes before using your brain."

The energy bar phenomenon capitalizes on a real human need—that of a convenient, nutrient-dense, concentrated food that travels well and doesn't spoil, and satisfies and tastes good.

Ignore the hype and advertising of the slick, packaged energy bars. These bars are not healthy food, they are candy bars - or worse - disguised as something the big food companies will tell you can substitute for meals, pump up your energy, or help you improve your athletic performance. There are better alternatives. Only REAL food will build up your body, fuel your energy and enhance your health. Stick to that which is unprocessed, unpackaged and has few ingredients. Your body will thank you for it.

# THAT WAS THE BAD.....

# *AND NOW FOR THE GOOD!*

# 13 Water

Adequate hydration is the foundation of optimal health. Among many other functions, fluid keeps our metabolism high, cushions our joints, enhances our mental alertness, and cleanses our body. General guidelines for fluid consumption are to consume half your body weight in ounces of water per day and make sure your urine is clear. If your urine is cloudy or apple-juice color, you are dehydrated! Consider the following:

* For many people, dehydration is mistaken as a hunger signal.
* Mild dehydration can slow the metabolism as much as three percent!
* One glass of water shuts down midnight "hunger" pains for many people.
* Dehydration is the foremost trigger of daytime fatigue.
* Eight to ten glasses per day can significantly ease joint and back pain.
* A two percent drop in body water can cause fuzzy short-term memory, trouble with basic math, and difficulty focusing on a computer screen or printed page.

Drinking five or more glasses of water per day significantly reduces the risk of developing cancer and other chronic diseases.

The sensation of thirst is triggered when 1.5 to 2.0 liters of water are already lost. If you are thirsty, you are dehydrated!

Seventy to seventy-five percent of muscle is fluid. Underhydration causes muscle shrinkage, and impairs athletic performance, metabolism, and body composition.

Athletes working intensely in hot weather can lose over 2.5 liters of water per hour!

# 14 High Quality Protein

*Grass-fed beef and bison, wild-caught fish, free-range chicken and whole (free-range) eggs*

With the obesity epidemic growing and the baby boomer generation aging, the benefits of high quality protein have never been more critical. Now, more than ever, it's important to re- think current dietary recommendations for high quality protein, and focus on achieving a level of protein intake to promote optimal health, not simply to meet the levels necessary to prevent protein deficiency.

The evidence suggests that increasing the proportion of protein in your diet will improve your body composition, help with weight loss and improve weight maintenance following weight loss.

Protein helps promote a feeling of fullness, and because it doesn't stimulate your insulin release, it can help prevent cravings for junky snacks. The claim that protein is a building block is very true. Protein is put to use by the body in building muscles, is stored for energy, and the amino acids are used throughout the body for various essential functions.

You may have noticed in recent years that a lot of health and fitness professionals argue over how much protein is necessary for good health, or to build muscle or lose weight. If you begin by increasing your daily protein intake beyond the Recommended Dietary Allowance (RDA) of 0.8 g/kg a day, you will find this may enhance muscle development and help to reduce progressive loss of muscle mass with age (sarcopenia). Most fitness experts go by the general rule of 1 gram of protein per pound of bodyweight per day (that would be over 2 grams of protein per kg of bodyweight per day). But this estimate has its flaws, as an obese individual would certainly never need extreme amounts of protein to equal 1 gram per pound of bodyweight.

In talking to fitness models, body builders

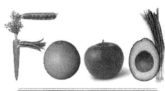

*for thought*

*Eating appropriate amounts of protein can help your body maintain the proper blood sugar levels and keep you from being hungry as often.*

and top athletes, we've found that one of the most important parts of their dietary regimen is protein intake. They all tend to eat a fairly high intake of protein. However, every body has its own unique needs and there is no magical ratio of protein that is "perfect" for you.

Besides creating a lean strong body, diets containing increased protein portions and reduced carbohydrates have positive effects in treating Type 2 diabetes, and reducing risk factors for coronary heart disease. So, not only does high-quality protein play an increasingly important role in weight management, muscle development and maintenance, but also disease prevention.

### *Selecting good quality protein is key to your body's ability to use it.*

High quality, grass-fed beef or bison, free-range chicken, organic eggs, and wild-caught fish are the most important types of protein to eat. They all contain the right ratios of good fats to bad fats and contain highly bio-available protein that is easier to digest than commercially raised livestock and poultry.

*If you're getting 20-30 grams of protein per meal from quality sources, and eating 5-6 small meals/day, that is going to provide all of the protein that most normal-sized people need.*

In addition, omega-3 fats in grass-fed meats and wild-caught fish are essential to optimal health and improve your cells' response to insulin, neurotransmitters and other messengers. They're also very important for the repair process when your cells are damaged. When your body is deprived of important essential fats like omega 3s, your metabolic rate slows down, so you can't burn calories as efficiently. In fact, weight gain is one of the symptoms of omega-3 deficiency.

In a recent research study, it was found that omega 3 fats helped to significantly decrease fat buildup in the heart and livers of obese rats. The study did not reveal the reasons why omega-3 fatty acids improved metabolic symptoms so much more, but the findings are in line with other studies that have also found superior health benefits from omega-3s. For more on the benefits of omega 3s, read chapter 16.

The best types of meat protein are not full of hormones, antibiotics and toxins; they are considered "clean" proteins, with no toxic residue to be stored in your tissues. Toxins stored in your body's fat will make it harder to lose that fat, once you start trying to change your diet. So stick to "clean" proteins with the highest quality protein you can get. Sure, it does cost a little more, but your body is utilizing more of the protein and getting loads more nutrition from it!

### *Grass-fed Beef or Bison (NOT the kind you get at the grocery store)*

Forget everything you've heard about beef - that it's high in saturated fat, that the best cuts are marbleized with fat and it's bad for you, that it increases your risk for certain diseases.

Red meat has gotten a bad reputation, but the truth is there is a healthier type of red meat than the commercially raised, grain-fed red meat you get from the grocery store.

Grass-fed beef and bison have more beta-carotene, Vitamin E and omega-3 fatty acids than beef produced using conventional cattle-feeding strategies. Grass-fed meat has been shown to aid in fat burning and muscle-building processes.

Three ounces of ground beef from regular grain-fed cattle contain about 40 micrograms of beta-carotene. In contrast, meat from cattle raised on grass has more than double the beta-carotene at 87 micrograms per three ounces of ground beef.

Beta-carotene is converted to Vitamin A in the body. Vitamin A is a critical fat-soluble vitamin that is important for vision, bone growth, reproduction, cell division and cell differentiation, and energy to burn calories.

In addition, meat from grass-fed animals is much higher in Vitamin E. Vitamin E is a fat-soluble vitamin with powerful antioxidant activity. Grass-fed cattle contain about three times as much Vitamin E per serving as grain-fed beef!

*Grass-fed meat is a far better choice, and is one of the best, most usable forms of high-quality fat-burning, muscle building proteins you can eat.*

The most important thing to remember about grass-fed cattle is the meat's fat content and the fat ratios. Not only does grass-fed beef have about thirty percent less fat per serving, but the healthy fats that it contains are highly beneficial and actually help you burn your body fat, to make you leaner and stronger.

Some fats are essential for losing weight and maintaining health. Your body needs a type of fat called essential fatty acids (EFAs) to function well; they must be obtained from the food that we eat. Grass-fed meat has significantly higher levels of the omega-3 essential fatty acids and conjugated linoleic acid (CLA) -- both known for their ability to help in fat burning, muscle building, and good general health, including possible benefits for cancer risk reduction, heart disease risk reduction, etc.

Meat from cattle raised on only grass have somewhere around sixty percent more omega-3 fatty acids, and a much better omega-6 to omega-3 ratio. Omega-3 fatty acids reduce inflammation and help prevent heart disease and arthritis. We need far more omega-3 fats and far less omega-6 fats than most people currently eat on a modern western diet. The latest research has linked higher blood levels of the omega-3 fatty acids, EPA and DHA, to lower rates of obesity.

These benefits are in addition to the fact that meat from grass-fed beef and bison is some of the highest quality protein that you can possibly eat—easily digestible and easily utilized by your body.

The large amounts of nutrients that grass fed cattle and bison consume in their daily diet are passed on to you. Besides omega-3 fatty acids and CLA, it also contains high amounts of Vitamins A and E, branch-chain amino acids (known for building lean muscle), digestive enzymes (so that this great protein is 100% utilized by your body), and essential nutrients that are known for their antioxidant properties.

And, grass-fed lamb and goat both have similar high-quality, usable protein as beef and bison. Ostrich meat and venison are some other healthy meats full of great nutrition, too.

As we mentioned in Part 1 of this book, another added benefit of meat from healthy, grass-fed animals is that dangerous E-coli does not thrive in a healthy, grass-fed animal! When cattle are fed a diet of grains, it increases the amount of acid in their stomachs during digestion. Increased acid and the drastic change in pH in cattle is the breeding ground for the dangerous E-coli bacteria that sickens so many people. Grass-fed cattle eat their natural diet, maintaining a balanced pH level, and the E-coli bacteria cannot grow in this environment. Why mess with Mother Nature? Grass fed meat is not only better for you, but safer too!

One of the best high protein snacks is pure, all-natural, grass-fed beef jerky. This is an easy and relatively inexpensive way to get good quality, lean protein when you just need a little something.

### Healthy Jerky Recipe
This is a fairly spicy recipe, so if you want it less spicy, cut the black pepper back to 1 Tbl or less. Use all organic ingredients and free range, grass fed beef or wild game (venison, elk, buffalo).

3 lbs of meat, sliced fairly thin
3/4 cup honey or brown sugar
1 Tbl Tabasco sauce

2 Tbl black pepper
2 Tbl garlic powder
4 bay leaves
1/3 cup sea salt
2 quarts of water

Heat mixture and pour over meat, making sure all meat pieces are covered. Cover pan and refrigerate for 24 hours. Put meat in a smoker and smoke until done (you can use a low-heat grill and smoker box). We like using hickory chips.

### Wild-Caught Fish

Like grass-fed meat, the fats in wild-caught fish are especially healthy. The BIG factor in both wild-caught fish and grass-fed meats is the type of fat and the fat ratios. Both have significantly higher levels of the essential fatty acid omega 3, which has powerfully positive effects in your body. The fat composition in farmed fish changes drastically when fed a grain-based diet and kept in pens, so stick to wild-caught fish. There is no comparison.

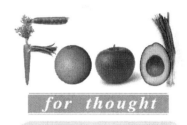

Wild caught fish to
choose:
*wild salmon*
*wild-caught halibut*
*wild cod*
*sardines*

Wild-caught fish, eating their natural diet, have the ideal fat composition—high in fat-burning, healthy omega 3s and low in inflammatory omega 6s. We know the benefits of omega 3s on our bodies, so eating wild caught fish seems to be the only choice.

Most of us know the healthy benefits that eating fatty fish or taking fish oil supplements provides to our heart, blood (cholesterol/triglycerides), brain, skin and joints. Well, add fat loss to those and the other numerous benefits, which are too long to list here.

What about mercury in fish? Mercury in fish occurs in some of the higher food chain predatory fish such as tuna and swordfish, so even though they are high in the good fats, they also store a considerable amount of mercury in that fat. Mercury has been shown to be very detrimental to the brain and overall health, and is a neurotoxin that is difficult for the body to eliminate.

What is the best type of wild-caught fish to eat? Everybody knows about salmon (wild salmon, of course, not farm raised) being a great source of omega-3 fatty acids and clean protein. Wild-caught halibut and wild cod are full of omega

3s as well.

Another great high omega-3 choice that doesn't have the issues with mercury is sardines. Before you think, "Eww, I don't like sardines!" it might be time to give them another look.

Sardines are a great choice for a quick, healthy meal - tons of muscle-building, appetite satisfying protein, super high in healthy omega 3 fats, and much lower in mercury and other pollutants than most fish.

One of the benefits of sardines is the long-chain omega-3 fats, such as EPA and DHA, which are far different from the shorter-chain, plant-based omega 3s like flaxseeds or walnuts. While full of other health benefits, such plant-based omega 3s are harder to convert into long-chain omega 3s in your body. One of the best ways to get the important EPA and DHA fats is through fatty wild-caught fish, fish oil, or krill oil.

The type of dietary fat (monounsaturated, saturated, or polyunsaturated) we consume alters the production of a group of biological compounds in our bodies known as eicosanoids. Eicosanoids have a significant biological influence on blood pressure, blood clotting, inflammation, immune function, and heart function. By eating enough omega-3 rich foods, you can help protect your health in many ways.

For example, one of the important things to remember about the inflammatory process is that it results in weight gain—or lack of ability to lose weight. So, reducing inflammation by eating enough healthy omega 3s is a key factor in fat loss!

Omega-3 oils also have additional protective effects against heart disease by:

  * Decreasing blood lipids (cholesterol, LDL and triglycerides)
  * Decreasing blood clotting factors in the vascular system
  * Increasing relaxation in larger arteries and other blood vessels
  * Decreasing inflammatory processes in blood vessels that can lead to
          plaque build up on arterial walls

Other studies have provided good news about the benefits of omega-3 oils for individuals with arthritis, psoriasis, ulcerative colitis, lupus, asthma, and certain cancers.

Most people with inflammatory health problems at some point have to resort to steroid-based drugs if they are not stringent about their diet. Steroids affect the body by causing immediate (and very difficult to lose) weight gain, facial puffiness and appetite increase. So avoiding having to resort to these heavy duty drugs will go a long way toward getting the lean, ripped body you are striving for!

Wild-caught fatty fish is also an excellent source of natural Vitamin E, a powerful antioxidant. Antioxidants, which also include Vitamin C and beta-carotene, deactivate harmful free radicals. Vitamin E also lowers the risk of heart disease by preventing the oxidation of low-density lipoproteins (LDLs or the "bad" cholesterol), and helping prevent buildup of plaque in coronary arteries.

As far as taste is concerned, there is no comparison. Wild fish almost always has a much better taste and texture, and it doesn't get the "fishy" smell and taste that farmed fish is known to have. Just keep in mind that wild-caught fish have a firmer texture and may be slightly drier, so be careful not to over cook.

## Free-range Chicken

Free-range chicken is becoming much more popular and easier to find. Not only is the taste much better, but the health benefits are much better than factory farm-raised chicken. Quite simply, free-range chickens make for healthier, better tasting meat. When animals are cared for properly, and given a supportive, all-natural environment in which to live, the food they yield is better for you and full of the nutrients you need.

The case for free-range chickens is becoming a stronger one for so many reasons, and we, the meat buying public, are becoming more and more health conscious and aware of its importance.

Most of us know about the antibiotics and hormones commercially-raised animals are given. They are fed hormone-enhanced grain and antibiotics, and fattened up as quickly as possible. The conditions under which such animals are raised play a large role as well. Commercially-raised chickens are raised in very close quarters where they can hardly move or turn around.

On the other hand, most free-range chickens do not need antibiotics or artificial growth hormones. They are allowed outside in their natural environment with sun and fresh air, and allowed to eat at will. Free-range chickens are allowed to live in large pens where they are highly mobile and stress free.

They are fed healthy, vegetarian feed, and are allowed to roam around and

*Keep some cooked chicken breasts on hand to throw into wraps with some lettuce and avocado for a delicious, quick and filling eat-on-the-run meal.*

eat greens, bugs, worms, and grubs. This is an important part of their natural diet. This increases the fat- burning omega 3s in their meat and their eggs. By eating more of their natural diet, their good fat ratios (omega-3 to omega-6) are kept in the healthy range.

Chicken meat has a naturally lower fat percentage than most red meats, but again it is best to purchase the free-range, organically raised kind. Otherwise, avoid eating the skin, which stores the largest amount of bad fats, hormones, antibiotics and other toxins.

### Whole Organic Free-range Eggs

Whole eggs including the yolk, not just egg whites, are an incredibly good source of usable protein. Most people know that eggs are one of the highest quality sources of protein. However, most people don't know that the egg yolks are the healthiest part of the egg. That's where almost all of the vitamins, minerals and antioxidants (such as lutein) are found.

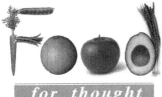

*Your best bet is to get eggs from a farmer or co-op where you know for certain that they allow the hens to graze freely outside for the majority of the day.*

Egg yolks contain more than ninety percent of the calcium, iron, phosphorus, zinc, thiamin, B6, folate, B12, and panthothenic acid of the egg. In addition, the yolks contain ALL of the fat-soluble Vitamins A, D, E, and K in the egg, as well as ALL of the essential fatty acids. Also, the protein of whole eggs is more bio-available than egg whites alone due to a more balanced amino acid profile that the yolks help to build.

Just make sure to choose free-range organic eggs instead of normal grocery store eggs. Similar to the grass-fed beef scenario, the nutrient content of the eggs and the balance between healthy omega-3 fatty acids and inflammatory omega-6 fatty acids (in excess) is controlled by the diet of the chickens.

Chickens that are allowed to roam free outside and eat a more natural diet will give you healthier, more nutrient-rich eggs with a healthier fat balance, compared with your typical grocery store eggs (that came from chickens fed only soy and corn, and crowded inside "egg factories" all day long).

Eggs from pastured free-range hens can contain ten times more omega-3 fatty acids than eggs from factory-farmed hens. Some companies may claim on the egg cartons that their hens are "free range," but this definition can be loosely interpreted by some companies that only let their hens outside for 5 or 10 minutes per day. This is a far cry from truly free-range, pastured hens that may spend most of their time outside in a given day.

If you can't find a co-op or farm near you, and you are forced to get your eggs from the grocery store, choose organic, free-range. In most instances, these will be higher quality eggs with more nutrition than typical factory-farmed eggs.

Eggs are such a versatile food; you can scramble them and throw in veggies to make an omelet, or boil to take with you for a great high-protein snack. Keep a few boiled eggs on hand to throw into a salad or sandwiches, or grated on top of soups or veggies. Throw an egg into your smoothie for added protein, or add egg to your stir- fry.

# 15 Going Raw

*Grass-fed raw dairy, milk and cheese*

Milk and dairy products sometimes get a bad rap. And rightly so, at least for the commercially produced kind. Hormones, antibiotics and white blood cells (left over from udder infections) all end up in the milk you buy from the grocery store. Once this kind of milk is extracted from the cow, it is then heated (pasteurized) to the point that many of the vital enzymes and nutrients are killed, and the milk proteins are distorted from the heat, so it is hard to digest and causes allergic reactions. It isn't much other than a white, fattening liquid at that point.

On the other hand, raw milk—especially milk from grass-fed cows - is a completely different story! Did you know that clean, raw milk from grass-fed cows was actually used as a medicine in the early part of the last century? Really! Milk straight from the udder, was used as medicine to treat some serious chronic diseases. From the time of Hippocrates to until just after World War II, this miracle food nourished and healed uncounted millions.

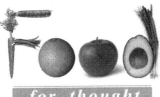

*for thought*

*Raw, unpasteurized, unhomogenized milk from grass-fed cows is the only source of cow's milk that can be considered healthy.*

Clean raw milk, cheese and butter from grass-fed cows are a complete and properly balanced food. You could live on it exclusively, if you had to. Raw dairy contains a wealth of healthy bodybuilding and fat-burning substances including: amino acids, enzymes, vitamins, minerals, and healthy fats such as CLA (conjugated linoleic acid).

Amino acids are the building blocks for protein, and we need somewhere around 20-22 of them for protein construction, which builds muscle. Raw dairy products have all 20 of the standard amino acids. About eighty percent of the proteins in milk are caseins, which are slow digesting, but easy to digest from raw milk. When pasteurized, they become hard to digest. The remaining twenty percent or so fall into the class of whey proteins, many of which have important physiological effects.

Also easy to digest, but very heat sensitive, are key enzymes and enzyme inhibitors, immunoglobulins (key immune factors), metal binding proteins, vitamin binding proteins and several growth factors.

Lactoferrin, an iron-binding protein found in raw milk, has numerous beneficial properties, including improved absorption and usage of iron, anti-cancer properties, and anti-microbial action against cavity-causing bacteria. Recent studies also reveal that Lactoferrin has powerful antiviral and antibacterial properties as well. So drinking a glass of raw milk is good for your teeth as well as the rest of your body.

CLA is abundant in milk from grass-fed cows. Among CLA's many potential benefits, it can help raise metabolic rate, gets rid of abdominal fat, boosts muscle growth, reduces resistance to insulin, strengthens the immune system and lowers food allergy reactions. Keep in mind, grass-fed, raw dairy has from three to five times the CLA amount found in the milk from feedlot cows (which produce the poor quality milk you buy at the grocery store)!

Raw milk also contains a broad selection of readily available vitamins and minerals, ranging from the familiar calcium and phosphorus, to Vitamins A and D, and trace elements. Raw, grass-fed dairy also contains a nutrient missing from our diets, called Vitamin K2. It is extremely valuable in helping the body absorb calcium, and therefore rebuilding bone, repairing cavities, and keeping the blood vessels clean. Only grass-fed dairy contains this important nutrient.

Two contributors in raw milk's antibiotic proteins and enzymes are lysozyme and lactoperoxidase. Lysozyme will break apart cell walls of some undesirable bacteria, while lactoperoxidase combines with other substances to help kill unwanted microbes. The immune enhancing components provide resistance to many viruses, bacteria and bacterial toxins. It may also help reduce the severity of asthma symptoms.

There are more than 60 functional enzymes in raw milk that perform an amazing amount of work. The most significant health benefit derived from food enzymes is the burden they take off the body in the digestion process and in assimilating nutrients.

Amylase, lactase, lipase and phosphatase in raw milk break down starch, lactose, fat (triglycerides) and phosphate compounds respectively, making milk more digestible and freeing up key minerals. Other enzymes, like catalase, lysozyme and lactoperoxidase help to protect milk from unwanted bacterial infection, making raw milk safe to drink.

What about the safety of raw milk? We have all been led to believe that milk MUST be pasteurized to kill bacteria and unwanted dangerous pathogens. Obviously, milk straight from a healthy cow's udder is clean. And a cow fed its natural diet and not pumped full of hormones and antibiotics will be a healthy cow, without illness, infections or an irritated udder.

Pasteurization of milk started way back in the early 1900s when unsanitary milking conditions were causing many to get sick. But raw milk has enzymes in it that actually kill off pathogens. Lactoferrin is one of these pathogen-killing enzymes in raw milk. In fact it is used to help sterilize beef processing plants. Raw milk contains very high levels of this enzyme-based pathogen killer. Pasteurization deactivates these enzymes that kill pathogens.

Other important enzymes that protect from bacteria are: xanthine oxidase, lactoperoxidase, lysozyme and nisin. All of these beneficial systems are destroyed by pasteurization. There are no remaining safety systems in processed pasteurized milk if harmful bacteria get into the pasteurized milk.

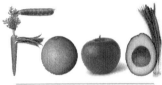

What about the stories of people getting sick from raw milk? These stories have proved to be not directly connected to the milk, but to other conditions unassociated with the milk. Sickly dairy cows, dirty conditions and unsanitary milking procedures are more likely the cause of bacteria in raw milk. Pasteurized milk actually has sickened thousands more than the reports of raw milk making people sick. The dairy industry and the huge industrialized dairy farms have fought to have raw milk made illegal, and many states now make it hard to obtain raw milk.

*www.RealMilk.com, www. Mercola.com, and www.westonaprice.org are three great resources for learning more about where to find co-ops and farms that sell raw milk in your area.*

What about cholesterol and saturated fat? Raw dairy contains about 3mg of cholesterol per gram - a decent amount. Our bodies make most of the cholesterol we need; that amount will fluctuate however, depending on what we get from food. Cholesterol in and of itself is not a harmful product, as we have been led to believe, but is a protective/repair substance. It's a waxy substance that our body uses as a building block for a number of key hormones. It's natural, normal, and essential, and it can be found in our brain, liver, nerves, blood, bile, and every cell membrane.

As for the fat in milk, two thirds of it is saturated. Saturated fats usually get blamed as the primary contributor to heart disease. Not so. Saturated fats play a number of key roles in our bodies, from construction of healthy cell membranes to key hormones that providing energy storage and padding for delicate organs, including the brain, to serving as a vehicle for important fat-soluble vitamins.

Fats also cause the stomach lining to secrete a hormone, which boosts production and secretion of digestive enzymes and signals the brain that we've eaten enough. With that trigger removed, non-fat dairy products and other fat-free foods can potentially contribute to over-eating.

One really important thing to note about raw, fresh milk—the taste! You have never tasted milk this delicious from a grocery store. Nothing tastes better. From the first try you will be hooked, even if you were not a big milk drinker before! There is absolutely no comparison between fresh raw milk and that thin, pasteurized, processed stuff you get from the grocery store.

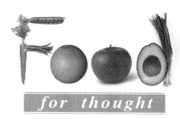

*Easier-to-find alternatives to raw cow's milk, especially suitable for those with dairy allergies or for vegans, are almond and coconut milks.*

Know the source of your raw milk and demand that it be from well-kept, grass-fed animals, and preferably organic. Raw milk is harder to find, as many states will not allow it to be sold commercially. Our advice is to avoid cow's milk altogether unless you can find a co-op or quality farm that sells raw milk from grass-fed cows.

# 16 The Good Fats

*Omega 3s, CLA, lard, grass-fed butter and coconut oil*

I t is good to incorporate a variety of healthy oils and fats into your diet. Together, they work as a team to supply your body with essential fatty acids for longevity, hormone balance, heart health, sharp vision, glowing moist skin and energy.

Twenty or so years ago, we all prudently switched our fat sources from butter and lard to margarine and Crisco®, due to the fact that doctors sounded the alarm that butter, lard and other saturated fats were primary contributors to heart disease and heart attacks.

What happened? Fast forward to today. We eat far less butter and lard than we did at the turn of the century, but heart disease has skyrocketed! Could the doctors be wrong? Yes.

New medical studies are surfacing showing it is not the cholesterol and saturated fats that we eat that contributes to heart attacks, but the trans fats like Crisco®, and highly processed omega-6 fats (soybean oil, sunflower oil, corn oil, safflower oil and other vegetable oils) that increase the inflammation that causes our bodies to send out cholesterol to mend the inflamed blood vessel walls.

## Omega 3s and CLAs

As mentioned in previous chapters, omega 3s are an extremely important essential fatty acid that humans do not get enough of in ratio to omega 6s. Eating grass-fed animals, along with free-range eggs and wild-caught fish can greatly improve our omega 3 intake without having to take supplements. Omega 3s offer a host of important benefits.

In a recent study, it was found that people with higher omega-3 blood levels had lower body mass indexes, narrower waists, and smaller hip circumferences.

The study suggests that omega 3 supplementation may play an important role in preventing weight gain and improving weight loss when supplemented within a structured weight-loss program.

Omega 3s may increase the burning of body fat by the process known as thermogenesis, in which oxidation of body fat burns it off in the form of body heat. These fatty acids also activate the enzymes responsible for burning fat, and combined with exercise, they increased the metabolic rate, which has an effect of burning more fat and losing weight.

One human study found that omega 3s boosted the feeling of fullness after a meal, among overweight and obese people participating in a weight loss program.

Several other studies have shown that eating foods with higher amounts of omega 3s combined with moderate exercise boosted fat loss and aided in increasing lean muscle.

Another key reason why omega-3 fatty acids have such a powerful effect on fat metabolism is that insulin levels are lowered when subjects are eating more omega 3s. By lowering insulin levels, it decreases the body's ability to store excess calories as fat—instead you burn fat!

In addition, omega 3 has many other positive benefits, including improving the skin's texture, lowering inflammation levels in the body, and helping autoimmune diseases. The omega 3s also reduce the risk of heart disease and stroke while helping to reduce symptoms of hypertension, depression, attention deficit hyperactivity disorder (ADHD), joint pain and arthritis, as well as certain skin ailments.

Some research has even shown that omega 3s boost the immune system and help protect the brain and nervous system from a variety of illnesses, including Alzheimer's disease, multiple sclerosis and cancer.

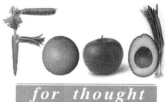

*for thought*

*Include organic, preferably grass-fed, butter, lard and extra virgin olive oil in your diet.*

The meat and milk, lard and beef-tallow from grass-fed cattle and bison, are also the richest known source of another type of good fat called "conjugated linoleic acid" or CLA— a much richer source than typical commercial beef. When cattle are raised on fresh pasture and no grains, their milk and meat contain as much as five times more CLA than products from animals fed conventional diets.

CLA has been proven in scientific studies in recent years to help in burning fat and building muscle (which means eating more of this type of healthy fat can help you get lean and ripped!).

In addition, CLA may be one of your most potent defenses against cancer. In studies, scientists have shown that CLA can lower an individual's risk for cancer and arteriosclerosis as well as reduce body fat and delay the onset of diabetes. So while it is making your body stronger and leaner, it is also protecting you from deadly diseases.

CLA has become so valued for its health benefits that many health food stores sell CLA supplements, but naturally-occurring CLA is metabolized more effectively and used better by the body than these synthetic supplements, which are prone to oxidation during shelf life.

### *The Benefits of Lard*

Lard is clearly winning the fat war over synthetic shortenings, like Crisco®. Forced on us over the last century, synthetic shortenings have proven to be a much bigger health hazard than lard because of the harmful trans fats they contain - the worst form of fats for our bodies.

Shortening surpassed lard in popularity fifty years ago when researchers connected animal fat in the diet to coronary heart disease. By the '90s, Americans moved to olive oil as the preferred oil, but shortening was still the solid fat to use over lard or even butter in far too many cookbooks and homes.

Now it can be argued that lard is good for you - in moderate doses of course! Lard's fat is also mostly monounsaturated. And even the saturated fat in lard has a neutral effect on blood cholesterol. Not to mention that lard has a higher smoking point than other fats, allowing foods like chicken to absorb less grease when fried in it.

And, of course, fat in general has a good side. The body converts it to fuel, which is then burned as a primary energy source, and it helps our bodies absorb nutrients, particularly calcium and fat-soluble Vitamins A, D, E and K. Keep in mind that lard or beef tallow should only come from grass-fed animals because they contain the higher quantities of the omega-3 fats and CLA.

### *Butter vs. Margarine*

If you are deciding whether to use butter or margarine, you're ALWAYS better off using butter. It is a real food with real benefits compared to the "fake food" margarine. Here are many of butter's healthy benefits:

* Butter contains CLA, a powerful fat burner, muscle builder, anti-cancer agent and immunity booster.
* Butter fat is a source of quick energy and great endurance energy.
* Butter contains the essential fatty acid Arachidonic Acid, which is an important muscle-building and fat-burning compound.
* Butter is a great source of Vitiman A. Butter contains the most easily absorbable form of Vitamin A, which among other things is good

for thyroid and adrenal health. Both are essential to fat burning and energy.

* Grass-fed butter contains the essential Vitamin K2; extremely essential in getting calcium in the bones and maintaining arterial health.

* Butter contains high levels of Vitamin D; essential to absorption of calcium, strengthening the immune system and overall feelings of wellbeing.

* Butter contains a substance called the "Wulzen Factor" or "Anti-Stiffness Factor" discovered by researcher Rosalind Wulzen. This compound protects against degenerative arthritis, hardening of the arteries, cataracts and calcification of the pineal gland. The Wulzen Factor is not present in the dairy products available in supermarkets, as it is destroyed by pasteurization.

* Butter contains the vital mineral selenium, which is a powerful cancer-fighting nutrient.

* Butter contains iodine in a highly absorbable form—highly recommended for adequate thyroid function and fat metabolism.

* Butter is a good source of lauric acid, important for your immune system, and also in treating fungal infections.

* Butter actually protects against tooth decay.

* Butter contains lecithin, which is essential for brain function and cholesterol metabolism.

* Butter contains anti-oxidants that protect against free radical damage.

Keep in mind that butter still is a highly concentrated source of calories, so be aware of controlling your portion sizes. However, since butter gives you nutrition that your body needs, it will help to reduce appetite and cravings, hence helping to control your caloric intake.

Similar to what we've discussed regarding other dairy products, the only source of healthy butter is from grass-fed cows. Once again, www.RealMilk.com can help you to find sources of raw, grass-fed dairy products near you. If you can't find butter from grass-fed cows, your next best bet is to find organic butter at your grocery store.

### *Coconut Oil: Another healthy saturated fat*

Coconut oil is often preferred by athletes, body builders and by those who are dieting. The reason behind this is that coconut oil is made up mostly of unique, healthy saturated fats called medium chain triglycerides (MCTs), which are easily converted into energy and are healthy for the heart and arteries. Coconut oil boosts energy and endurance, and enhances the athletic performance.

Coconut oil has positive benefits in reducing body fat. It contains short and medium-chain fatty acids that can rev up the body's metabolism. It is also easy to digest and aids the healthy functioning of the thyroid (critical to metabolism and weight loss) and enzyme systems. It also increases the body's metabolism by removing stress on the pancreas, which means the body will have a bigger supply of energy to burn body fat.

People who live in tropical coastal areas and eat coconut oil daily as a primary cooking oil are normally not overweight. Pure coconut oil (make sure it is not hydrogenated) is actually one of the best options for a cooking oil, due to its highly stable nature under heat. This makes it much less inflammatory to your body compared to other oils such as soybean oil, corn oil, or other "vegetable" oils.

Fats have come full circle; we are now reverting back to the good traditional fats that our ancestors have cooked with for years. Long before heart disease, cancer and other serious diseases appeared, these fats were used in abundance. Now we are beginning to realize they are not the bad guys they have been made out to be. So enjoy your butter, coconut oil and lard (in small doses) and feel good about it!

# 17 Nuts

*Walnuts, almonds, cashews, pecans, macadamia, pistachios*

A high-fat food that's good for your health and helps you lose weight? Yes! Forget about shying away from nuts and put them at the top of your list of healthy, lean-body snacks!

Several studies have shown that dieters who include reasonable amounts of nuts in their diet actually lose more weight than those who do not eat nuts. Nuts are the perfect snack. As long as you can restrain yourself from overeating, nuts can actually be fat-fighters and help with weight loss.

Protein and fat in nuts help you feel fuller and stop cravings. Since nuts have no sugars they do not promote an insulin response, which means they are more likely to be used as energy, and they will not stimulate your appetite like a starchy or sweet food will. Nuts will not put you on that merry-go-round of eating, hunger, more eating, and weight gain.

Nuts will help maintain higher levels of fat-burning hormones in your body as well as help control appetite and cravings so that you essentially eat less calories overall, even though you're consuming a high-fat food.

Besides their lean body benefits, nuts are a highly nutritious food to include in your diet. Most nuts are high in monounsaturated fats, the same type of health-promoting fats as are found in olive oil, which have been associated with reduced risk of heart disease and cancer. Nuts also contain polyunsaturated fats, healthy saturated fats, and linoleic acid, another healthy fat that the body utilizes for essential fatty acids. Eating controlled amounts of healthy fats can satisfy your cravings and keep you from over-indulging in something far unhealthier, like hunger-producing starchy, sweet, fattening carbs.

Nuts have loads of great nutrition, although their fat content (75 to 95 percent of total calories) means you shouldn't eat a zillion at one time. And really, because they are so satisfying to your appetite, you probably won't.

Macadamia, the gourmet of nuts, is the highest in healthy fats. Walnuts, Brazil nuts and pine nuts also have additional health benefits because they're rich in omega-3 fatty acids.

Five significant, human research studies all found that nut consumption is linked to a lower risk for heart disease. Researchers who studied data from the Nurses Health Study estimated that substituting nuts for an equivalent amount of carbohydrates in an average diet resulted in a thirty percent reduction in heart disease risk. Nuts contain significant amounts of Vitamin E. As an antioxidant, Vitamin E can help prevent the oxidation of LDL cholesterol, which can damage arteries.

Nuts are chockfull of hard-to-get minerals, such as copper, iron, magnesium, manganese, zinc and selenium. Iron helps your blood deliver oxygen to your muscles and brain, while zinc helps boost your immune system and brain function. Selenium is a potent cancer-fighting mineral, and aids the thyroid gland, which regulates metabolism and fat-burning in the body.

Potassium is an important electrolyte involved in nerve transmission, heart function and blood pressure. Nuts are good for your cardiovascular health by providing 257 mg of potassium and only trace amounts of sodium (that's if you eat the unsalted kind!), making them an especially good choice to in protecting against high blood pressure and atherosclerosis.

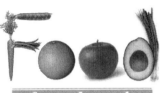

*Almonds and walnuts top the list in nutrition, but other nuts are healthy, too, including pistachios, pecans, cashews, and - even though they are actually a legume - peanuts.*

Magnesium is nature's vaso-dilator. When your body has enough magnesium, veins and arteries relax and dilate, which lessens resistance and improves the flow of blood, oxygen and nutrients throughout the body. This lowers your blood pressure as well as having an overall relaxing effect. Magnesium has been shown as essential for prevention of heart attacks.

Nuts are also a good source of fiber and protein, which of course helps to control blood sugar and can aid in weight loss.

While all nuts are healthy, there a few superstars:

***Brazil nuts*** contain a very high amount of selenium; about 70 to 90 micrograms per nut. So just 3 or 4 Brazil nuts will provide you with ample amounts of this essential nutrient. And, nuts do their part to keep bones strong by providing magnesium, manganese, and boron, essential for bone health.

In addition to healthy fats and Vitamin E, a quarter cup of almonds contains almost 99 mg of magnesium (that's 25percent of the daily value for this important mineral), plus 257 mg of potassium.

***Walnuts, pecans and chestnuts*** have the highest antioxidant content of the tree nuts, with walnuts winning out over the others in antioxidant content. Pecans are effective in preventing prostate enlargement and prostate cancer in men. And peanuts (although technically a legume) also contribute significantly to our dietary intake of antioxidants. Many other nuts are missing the amino acid lysine, but peanuts are rich in lysine and antioxidant polyphenols, like those found in berries. They also provide the most complete protein.

*Pistachios* help to reduce the risk of macular degeneration, a common cause of visual loss in older individuals. Pistachios contain two important carotenoids, lutein and zeaxanthin, compounds which help prevent this common eye condition. Carotenoids are also strong antioxidants that help to offset cell injury and damage. A daily snack of pistachios could be a tasty and effective way to protect one of your most important senses - your vision. Pistachios are also high in protein, making a satisfying snack.

The list of health benefits attached to each individual nut is endless. Other nuts that are particularly good include: hazelnuts because they are one of the richest sources of the antioxidant Vitamin E; and cashews for their high iron content, which is needed to make hemoglobin - the red pigment in the blood.

Go for raw nuts or raw nut butters instead of roasted nuts if you can; it helps to maintain the quality and nutritional content of the healthy fats that you will eat. Remember that polyunsaturated fats are unstable and become inflammatory to your body when they've been exposed to heat, so roasted nuts are not the best option. Stay away from the commercially prepared roasted and salted nuts, as these often have unhealthy cottonseed or soybean oils added, thus canceling out many of the healthy effects of the nuts.

And for an added change, try almond butter, cashew butter, pecan butter, or macadamia butter to add variety to your diet and make it easier to get more of the quality nutrition of nuts into your diet.

Here's a blood sugar balancing, heart-healthy, delicious way to include nuts in your diet.

### *Nutty Energy Snack* - **Power balls**

40 dates (About a package and a half)
1/2 c raw almonds
1/2 c raw cashews
1/2 c crunchy peanut or almond butter
1/2 c ground flax
1/2 to 3/4 cup dried blueberries
3-4 Tbs green powder

4 Tbs cinnamon

Place nuts and flax in food processor, process till nuts are well ground. Add remaining ingredients and process until mixture forms a ball. (You can adjust the ingredients to taste.)

Roll into 1" balls, then roll in unsweetened coconut. I use a mini cookie scoop to portion out the balls. These store well in an airtight container.

# 18 Avocados

A vocados are another so-called "fatty food" that many of us have been conditioned to avoid, but this is a power-packed super food! Not only is this fruit super high in monounsaturated fat, but also chock full of vitamins, minerals, micronutrients, and antioxidants.

The healthy fats and other nutrition you get from avocados helps your body to maintain proper levels of hormones that help with fat loss and muscle building. The healthy fat content in avocados helps control insulin levels, makes you feel full longer and takes away junk food cravings. And that equals a leaner, healthier body. Avocados are a great snack!

Avocados contain plenty of oleic acid, a monounsaturated fat that helps lower cholesterol and is helpful in preventing breast cancer and other cancers. Avocados are also a good source of potassium, a mineral that helps regulate blood pressure. Adequate intake of potassium can help guard against circulatory diseases, like high blood pressure, heart disease or stroke.

One cup of avocado has about a quarter of your required daily amount of folate, or folic acid, a B vitamin that plays an essential role in making new cells by helping to produce DNA and RNA. Folate also helps lower the risk of birth defects in babies, and is important for heart health. One study showed that individuals who consume folate-rich diets have a much lower risk of cardiovascular disease or stroke than those who do not consume as much of this vital nutrient.

Avocados are also a very concentrated dietary source of the carotenoid lutein which is good for eye health. It also contains measurable amounts of related carotenoids (zeaxanthin, alpha-carotene and beta-carotene) plus significant quantities of tocopherols (Vitamin E), all significant cancer fighting ingredients.

Since avocados contain a large variety of nutrients, including vitamins, minerals as well as great healthy fat, enjoying a few slices of avocado in your tossed salad, or mixing some chopped avocado into your favorite salsa will not only add a rich, creamy flavor, but will greatly increase your body's ability to absorb the healthy carotenoids that vegetables provide.

Cut up fresh avocados in your salad; add to sandwiches, omelets, or Mexican food. Guacamole (mashed avocados with garlic, onion, tomato, pepper, etc) is a super delicious and nutritious satisfying snack. Avoid the fattening corn chips and dip veggies in your guacamole instead, or eat with a fork or spread on sandwiches or a juicy grass- fed hamburger. There are a zillion delicious ways to enjoy avocados!

Avocados are best when firm but yield slightly to touch.

# 19 Organic Berries

*Blueberries, acai, goji, strawberries, raspberries and more*

Berries contain a healthy dose of fiber, which slows your carbohydrate absorption and digestion, and controls blood sugar levels to help prevent insulin spikes, making berries a great superfood for fat loss and a lean body!

A cup of strawberries contains over 100 mg of Vitamin C, which is better than orange juice. Vitamin C strengthens the immune system and helps build strong, connective tissue. Strawberries contain calcium, magnesium, folate and potassium, and have very few calories. If they are available, organic strawberries are far superior than non-organic, and are well worth the extra price.

Non-organic strawberries are one of the highest sprayed crops, and since strawberries really have no skin or rind, they soak up all those pesticides and herbicides. Even washing won't get rid of that.

One cup of blueberries offers a smaller amount of Vitamin C, but high amounts of minerals and phytochemicals and very low calories. Blueberries are also extremely high in antioxidants. The same amount of cranberries is similar. One cup of raspberries offers Vitamin C and potassium.

You can choose other berries with similar power-packed nutrition, such as loganberries, currants, gooseberries, lingonberries and bilberries.

The pigments in berries that create the bright colors are also good for your health. Berries contain potent phytochemicals and flavonoids that may help to prevent cancer, reduce heart disease risk, and protect skin from damage. Blueberries and raspberries also contain lutein, which is important for healthy vision.

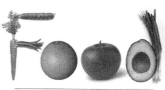

*for thought*

*Berries - including blueberries, strawberries, raspberries, and even the "exotic" goji berry and acai berry - are powerhouses of nutrition... packed with vitamins and minerals, and also some of the best sources of antioxidants of any food in existence.*

Every grocery store carries a wide variety of fresh and frozen berries. Look for ripe, colorful and firm berries with no sign of mold or mushy spots. Berries can also be found in the frozen section of the grocery store. Once they thaw, they will not be as firm as freshly picked berries, but they are still delicious and good for you. Throwing them into the blender for a smoothie is a great way to enjoy frozen berries in the winter.

For the freshest berries, try farmers' markets that offer local berries harvested that same day. Some berry farms allow you to pick your own berries. Nothing is better than picking and eating berries warm from the sun and bursting with freshness and nutrients!

### *Very Berry Smoothie*

Our very favorite, easy berry smoothie can be made with:

1or so cups of frozen berries

1 banana

1 scoop of your favorite protein powder (or if you don't have protein powder, throw in a raw egg-its perfect protein)

1/2 cup of orange juice or any other juice you have

A few ice cubes

Blend together all ingredients. These are delicious and nutritious, and the protein makes them a satisfying meal or snack. Don't worry about the raw egg— raw eggs are fine as long as the shell is not cracked. And if you're using fresh farm eggs instead of the grocery store kind, they are even safer. Rinse them off before using.

# 20 Organic Dark Leafy Greens

*Salad greens, quick-cooking greens, hearty greens*

D id you know our ancient ancestors used to eat up to six pounds of vegetation per day? As they traveled, they picked and ate green leaves as they went. That's like eating a grocery bag full of greens every day! Very few of us even get the minimum of three cups a week! And yet, these leafy greens deliver a bonanza of vitamins, minerals, fiber, antioxidants, and phytonutrients!

Leafy vegetables are the ideal lean body food, as they are typically very low in calories. They are useful in reducing the risk of cancer and heart disease since they are low in fat, high in dietary fiber, and rich in folic acid, Vitamins K, C, E, and many of the B vitamins, iron, calcium, potassium and magnesium as well as contain a host of phytochemicals.

Did you know that eating three or more servings a week of green leafy vegetables significantly reduces the risk of stomach cancer, the fourth most frequent cancer in the world? Cabbage, cauliflower, Brussels sprouts, and broccoli are rich in natural chemicals called indoles and isothiocyanates, which protect against colon and other cancers. And broccoli sprouts contain 10 times as much sulforaphane, a cancer-protective substance, than does mature broccoli, and are extremely powerful weapons in fighting cancer.

Dark green leafy vegetables are, for being low calorie, one of the most concentrated sources of nutrition of any food. They also provide a variety of phytonutrients including beta-carotene, lutein, and zeaxanthin, which protect our cells from damage and our eyes from macular degeneration and cataracts, among other benefits. Dark green leaves even contain small amounts of healthy omega-3 fats.

The superstar nutrient here is Vitamin K. A cup of most cooked greens provides at least nine times the minimum recommended intake of Vitamin K, and even a couple cups of dark green leafy salad greens will give you the minimum all on their own. Recent research has provided evidence that this vitamin may be even more important than we once thought (the current minimum may not be optimal), and many people do not get enough of it.

Some of the fantastic benefits of Vitamin K:

* Regulates blood clotting
* Puts calcium in the bones, not in the bloodstream
* May help prevent and possibly even reduce atherosclerosis by
    reducing calcium in arterial plaques
* May be a key regulator of inflammation, and may help protect us
    from inflammatory diseases including arthritis
* Vitamin K is a fat-soluble vitamin, so make sure to use a dressing with
    healthy fats (such as extra virgin olive oil or Udo's Choice Oil
    blend) on your salad, or add avocado slices to your salad. Adding
    a small amount of butter or cheese to cooked veggies can also help
    with vitamin absorption.

Greens have very little carbohydrates, but lots of fiber, which make them slower to digest. So, greens have very little impact on blood glucose. In some diets, greens are even treated as a "freebie," carb-wise (meaning the carbohydrate doesn't have to be counted at all). All of this equates to lean, mean nutrition!

Greens can be categorized into three different groups, depending on how you prepare them:

*Salad greens*—These are usually eaten raw. In general, the darker the color, the more nutritious. Iceberg lettuce, for example, is extremely low in nutrients, and is virtually worthless nutritionally. Lettuce's more colorful family members are much more worthy of your attention. For example, romaine lettuce, red leaf lettuce, bib lettuce, and baby greens have eight times the Vitamin A and six times the Vitamin C as iceberg lettuce. Bib lettuce and red and green leaf lettuce make great substitutes for bread too. Try a tuna salad, or any of your other favorite sandwiches, wrapped in lettuce instead of bread.

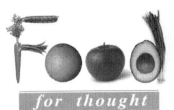

*Chop up the stems of chard and put them in tuna salad instead of celery. If you haven't tried chard, you really should - you may be pleasantly surprised!*

When you have a choice, a variety of greens is always best as each has its own constellation of nutrients. Go for as many different colors and shades of green as you can! One of the best choices is baby greens. These tender leaves usually come in a wide variety of types and colors, each with its own treasure trove of nutrients, and what's more - they are delicious!

Green, leafy vegetables provide a great variety of colors from the dark bluish-green of kale to the bright green of spinach. Leafy greens run the whole gamut of flavors, from sweet and nutty to bitter; from peppery to earthy. Young plants generally have small, tender leaves and a mild flavor. Many mature plants have tougher leaves and stronger flavors. Try Mache and baby Arugula. Arugula is a healthy topper to grass-fed burgers or side dish with omelets. Arugula has a super-high nutrient density and a delicious nutty, spicy flavor!

*Quick-cooking greens*—These can either be eaten raw or lightly cooked. Spinach is the best-known example in this category. It takes only seconds to cook a spinach leaf; overcooked spinach is not very tasty. Most quick-cooking greens take just a few minutes to cook—and should not be overcooked or they become mushy and tasteless.

Cooked greens shrink quickly so you can get lots of nutrition from them. Six cups of raw greens become approximately one cup of cooked greens.

Swiss chard is a quick-cooking green that also can be eaten raw, though it isn't usually. Chard is now available in many colors, which are often milder-

*How to Cook Greens: Greens can be braised (cooked fairly slowly in a small amount of liquid, usually a flavorful stock), sautéed (cooked quickly in a small amount of oil), or a combination of the two. They can also be steamed or boiled, but most people like to add some other flavors that go well with greens, like chopped fresh garlic, small bits of cooked bacon, lemon, vinegar, hot chilies, anchovies, or onion. Just remember that greens taste best when they are very lightly cooked. Take them off the heat when they are just limp, but still bright green.*

tasting than the more traditional chard. Chard and spinach are good places to start with cooked greens, as they are easy, and not as bitter as some others. Beet greens are also quick-cooking (and delicious), and are actually related to chard and spinach. Escarole, dandelion greens and sorrel are also relatively quick-cooking greens.

*Hearty Greens*--Many people seem to have a deep-seated fear of kale and collard greens (at least outside the southern U.S.), but I encourage you to give them a try, as they have the most nutritional benefits of all. Over time, they may even become favorites.

Kale and collard greens are the most common examples of hearty greens. They do require cooking, although not as much as many people think. Yes, you can cook collards for an hour, but if you cut the greens from the fibrous stems they can be tender in 10-15 minutes. Same is true for kale.

Greens can also be thrown into almost any soup or skillet dish, or even omelets, especially the milder-tasting greens such as chard.

# 21 Healthy Sweeteners

*Real maple syrup, raw honey,
raw agave nectar and stevia*

Our craving for sweets often ruins the most well-intentioned lean body plan, and we succumb to chocolates, handfuls of cookies, a slice of cake, a generous scoop of ice cream, or other such decadent fare. The key ingredient in all of these items, and in essentially most of the sweets available on the market, is sugar or worse - high- fructose corn syrup.

Too much sugar is often the culprit in sabotaging our diets, but it seems hard to avoid or resist. Sometimes you just crave a little something sweet. Artificial sweeteners are loaded into so many foods and snacks promoted as "diet" foods, but the long-term negative health aspects as well as the potential weight gain is good enough reason for you to avoid any and all artificial sweeteners.

Fortunately there are a variety of natural sweeteners that have been quite common in supermarkets for a very long time, and are likely sitting on your shelf in your pantry at this very moment.

Honey makes an excellent alternative to sugar and has some health benefits for you compared to refined sugar. Although honey is still a form of sugar (be aware of its caloric impact), one benefit of honey over refined sugar is that, according to several studies, raw honey can actually improve your body's ability to process glucose. On the other hand, refined sugar negatively affects your body's ability to process glucose over time.

Different types of honey contain different nutrients and health benefits, depending on types of pollen and flowers the honey comes from. All honey possesses antibacterial agents and acts as an antioxidant. Honey contains Vitamins B2 and B6, and is a good source of iron. Consuming just a spoonful of honey each day can raise the antioxidant levels in our bodies, and it is also the healthiest natural sweetener available for those with Type 2 diabetes. Raw honey can often be found at Whole Foods, local farm stands, and even some grocery stores, and is by far the best you can get - chock full of enzymes as well as the above listed nutrients.

Honey is a great replacement for sugar in many recipes, and because it is quite a bit sweeter, you can use a smaller amount. The rule of thumb is about a 1/2 cup of honey per cup of sugar. Also, when cooking you should reduce liquids in the recipe by a 1/4 cup to ensure proper consistency. Honey also serves to brown foods more easily as they cook, so cooking temperatures should be lowered by 25°F.

Maple syrup is another product many of us have in the home, and is another natural sweetener that can often be used in place of sugar. We are talking about real, pure, natural maple syrup—not Aunt Jemima® (which is just flavored corn syrup)! Real maple syrup is a good source of minerals and trace nutrients. As with honey, maple syrup is also a useful antioxidant, and possesses a good amount of zinc, which can help prevent atherosclerosis and lower cholesterol as well as strengthen the immune system.

Maple syrup can be purchased in three specific colors or grades, each denoting a particular flavor. The lighter syrups (Grade A) will possess a more subtle flavor, while the darkest coloring (Grade B or C) yields the strongest, sweetest flavor. The darker maple syrups typically contain higher antioxidant and nutrient levels than Grade A maple syrup.

As with honey, you need to be aware of the high caloric level of maple syrup, as it is still a concentrated source of sugar. However, it is definitely a better choice than refined sugar.

Even though honey and maple syrup are slightly healthier options compared to refined white sugar, your best bet is still to reduce your dependence on added sweeteners to food and drinks by learning to adjust your taste buds to prefer less sweetness.

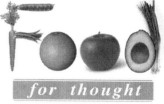

*for thought*

*Use just a tiny pour of real maple syrup in your coffee instead of white sugar. For teas, try a small dab of raw honey. Maple syrup also is great on oatmeal.*

Agave nectar is the nectar of a cactus and can be used anywhere you may use syrup. It has a low glycemic index, so is a good, natural sweetener for those with diabetes.

Blackstrap molasses is another option for a natural sweetener that can be used in baking. It is a particular type of molasses that is rich in several essential vitamins and minerals, including a good concentration of manganese, iron, calcium, potassium, and more. It is also substantially lower in calories than other natural sweeteners.

Because molasses has a such a distinctive flavor, it may not be used as often as other natural sweeteners as a replacement for sugar, but it can enhance some foods, such as baked beans and gingerbread, with unique flavors.

Newer low or no-calorie sweeteners are starting to hit the mainstream. The healthiest of these is stevia. Stevia comes from the leaves of a shrub native to Paraguay and Brazil, and has been used as a sweetener for many years in South America. Stevia is about three hundred times sweeter than sugar, and has all the benefits of a sweetener without being bad for you - or fattening. It's truly natural (not some chemical compound from a laboratory), free of calories, doesn't promote tooth decay, and won't elevate blood sugar levels or cause weight gain.

To sugar-crazy and diet-conscious Americans, stevia should be incredibly popular and well known, but up until recently, it was not allowed in food or easily found. The Food and Drug Administration (FDA) banned stevia in 1991. Why? Like many proponents of stevia, the sugar industry has a hand in the FDA's strict stance. The FDA ban allowed it to be sold only as a dietary "supplement,"and it could only be found in health food stores in the supplement aisle, right next to the vitamins. It was pretty difficult to find, and never in the sugar or sweetener aisle - until now.

In the many years that stevia has been used in South America and Japan, no ill health effects have ever been attributed to its use. Like all the previous low-calorie sweeteners out there, there have been some conflicting stories on the health benefits and safety of stevia, but it has been approved by the FDA as a general-purpose sweetener since December 2008.

The actual name of the plant is stevia. Stevia's sweetness comes from its leaves. The stevia leaves are milled, and a freshwater brewing method is used to extract the sweetness. This extract is then purified further until a very high purity Reb-A (Rebaudiosides A) is obtained. The stevia plant also contains the sweeteners Reb- B, C, D and E, dulcoside A, and steviolbioside.

Just this year, U.S.-based beverage giants PepsiCo and Coca-Cola reported they were looking to switch from (or at least offer customers the choice of) Splenda® to Reb-A.

"We're testing stevia and Reb-A in a variety of products, but it absolutely comes down to taste," said Joe Tripodi, chief marketing officer for Coca-Cola.

In 2005, Coca-Cola and the food giant Cargill began to work on their own form of the sweetener. The companies are now marketing their stevia sweetener as Truvia®. You may see food items now sweetened with Truvia®. Coca-Cola is initially using it in two of its Odwalla juice drinks and in the new Sprite Green.

PepsiCo's stevia sweetener is being marketed as PureVia®, and like Truvia®, the marketing is pushing the fact that it is natural.

"This is a potential game-changer among zero-calorie sweeteners," said

Lou Imbrogno, PepsiCo's senior vice president of Pepsi Worldwide Technical Operations, at a press conference in July 2008. PepsiCo's partner is using stevia in its Sobe Lifewater® drinks and in a new line of Tropicana® Orange Juice, Trop50.

Stevia is the standout sweetener in the marketplace because it is what the public is looking for in a low-calorie sweetener to replace the questionable and not-so-natural Splenda® and NutraSweet® chemically-derived, artificial sweeteners.

Splenda®'s creator, McNeil Nutritionals, is getting in on the stevia craze as well. In March 2010, Sun Crystals All-Natural Sweetener® was launched, which combines stevia with pure cane sugar. This will be marketed as being as natural as sugar with half the calories.

NutraSweet® has reported that they were not worried about stevia. But coincidentally, the company is working on its own NutraSweet Natural® made with stevia! At least now they can compete head-to-head with stevia in the market.

While the many chemically-processed artificial sweeteners have been connected to lung tumors, breast tumors, and other rare types of tumors, several forms of leukemia, and chronic respiratory disease in several rodent studies as well as rashes, headaches, and other serious and nasty side effects, stevia, Reb-A and its derivatives seem to be the safest of all low-calorie sweeteners for the moment.

*You can find stevia blends for your own use at this site: http://www. Naturally-Stevia.com*

Try stevia in your favorite beverages like coffee, tea, lemonade, and more. Depending on the brand and type of stevia you use, the taste may vary. Some of the health food store varieties had a "green" aftertaste, but really not bad—just something to get used to. Now that stevia is becoming more mainstream, the taste has improved. And some stevia comes in liquid form with great flavors like vanilla, toffee, lemon, etc. Give it a try!

# 22 Healthy REAL Food Energy Bars

Whether out on a mega-mile bike ride, running, or just on the run, occasionally you need to have something on hand for a quick and healthy snack. While "energy bars" are marketed this way, many are deceiving in that they are actually just glorified candy bars full of sugar, corn syrup and artificial ingredients—nothing our bodies really need, especially if we want them to be lean, healthy and strong.

However, there are a few really good energy bars out there. They may not be as easy to find, but when you do find them, these bars are worth stocking up on. Look for a short list of all natural ingredients, low sugar, and a genuine protein source like whey or nuts, as opposed to soy isolates. Here are some suggestions:

* Raw Revolution®
* Organic Food Bars®
* Larabars®
* Prograde Cravers®
* Boomi Bar®

*Raw Revolution*® – This is an organic, live food bar with sprouted flax seeds, based on the principle that raw foods have higher nutrient content than cooked foods. These are some of the best tasting bars in the industry and come in flavors like Raspberry & Chocolate, Spirulina & Cashew, Cashew & Agave Nectar, Hazelnut & Coconut, and Tropical Mango, just to name a few.

*Organic Food Bars*® - This is actually the brand name. Depending on which flavor, these are usually a base of organic almond butter (or cashew butter) with a certain type of fruit, organic seeds, organic biosprouts (quinoa, etc), and some organic rice protein. Some flavors include an organic dark chocolate as well. They also have a line of bars that use exclusively raw ingredients.

Not only are these food bars extremely nutritious, but delicious as well. Flavors to choose from include: blueberry, cranberry, chocolate chip, high protein, and more.

*Larabars*® - These are even simpler in ingredients than the Organic Food Bars. Larabar is a delicious blend of unsweetened fruits, nuts and spices - energy in its purest form. Made from 100 percent whole food, each flavor contains no more than eight ingredients, but most flavors only have two or three ingredients. They are sweet, with no added sweeteners, and sustaining, with no added fillers, supplements or flavorings. Just real, whole food loaded with nature's own minerals and vitamins.

All of the vitamins, minerals, fiber, protein, good carbohydrates and healthy fats are uncooked and unprocessed. They are gluten-free, dairy free, soy free, vegan, and kosher. The essential enzymes, which are necessary for the digestion and utilization of nutrients, remain completely intact in their most natural effective state. A diet abundant in raw, unprocessed foods is important for health and longevity.

Some of the flavors are: coconut cream pie, chocolate mole, chocolate coconut, cherry pie, apple pie, ginger snap and more.

*Prograde Cravers*® - These are made by Prograde Nutrition. These are definitely some of the tastiest nutrition bars around. (Try the peanut butter flavor!) They are also made with all organic ingredients using nut butters, rice protein, organic dark chocolate, etc. These aren't available in stores, and you can only find these organic bars online at: **http://natural.getprograde.com/cravers.**

*Boomi Bar*® – These bars are sweetened with honey, all natural, and contain primarily nuts and fruit. There are several different, delicious flavors to choose from. For example, the Macadamia Paradise bar contains: madacamia nuts, pineapple, honey, raisin, sesame seeds, puffed amaranth, crisped rice and salt.

The healthy nutrition bars listed here make great quick snacks while you're traveling, while at work, or any time you just need a quick pick-me-up energy bar.

Carry some with you or in your car, just to make sure there are healthy options to choose when you are ravenous. That way you won't be as tempted by fast food joints or junk food vending machines.

Stores like Whole Foods have other whole, raw healthy energy bars as well, like Jay Robb Bars®, Perfect Food Bars®, Greens Plus Omega 3®, Chia Bars®, Bliss® bars and others. Even some grocery stores are beginning to carry wider choices.

Just be sure to avoid processed ingredients like refined flours, soy protein, and a lot of sugars, and choose the bars with easily identifiable and NATURAL ingredients. Be aware that at typical chain grocery stores, mega-stores like Wal-Mart and most convenient stores, 99 percent of the bars sold are usually made with soy protein, chemical additives, and loads of sweeteners.

# 23 Dark Chocolate

One of the major reasons diets and other weight loss programs fail is because you end up feeling deprived. Life isn't about that. It's about changing your bad habits, and indulging in small amounts, once in a while. Integrating chocolate and other foods you enjoy, in small doses, can help you make your new lean and mean diet plan successful and easy to incorporate into your daily life--without feeling deprived!

Every once in a while you need a sweet, satisfying treat, and chocolate seems to fit the bill. Chocolate is actually good for you, but it can't be just any old chocolate you grab off the shelf. No M&Ms® or a big ol' Hershey® bar! That's just cheap chocolate with lower levels of actual cocoa and higher levels of refined sugar and other junk.

Occasional chocolate treats are not of any great importance, if you are doing everything else right. One or two small pieces of dark chocolate will not ruin your diet. In fact, knowing that you can allow yourself a treat or reward for sticking to a lean, healthy diet can make those dietary changes a lot easier to live with. And dark chocolate is good for you!

Keep in mind that milk chocolate and white chocolate don't offer the same health benefits as dark chocolate. Look for good quality dark, organic chocolate, with few ingredients, in the health food section of your grocery store or at a place like Whole Foods or Trader Joe's. These stores carry a wide selection of dark, delicious, organic chocolate with yummy additions like nuts, dried fruits and other scrumptious flavors.

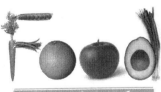

*Look for dark chocolate with a cocoa content of at least 70 percent or higher to keep your sugar content low.*

Any good dark chocolate will list the cocoa content on the package. Generally, chocolates in the range of 70-80 percent cocoa content have the best taste but have much lower sugar levels than milk chocolate or dark chocolates that are lower than 70 percent cocoa. Many milk chocolates are only 30 percent cocoa, and some cheap dark chocolates are only 50 percent cocoa. This means that the remaining non-cocoa ingredients are sugar and other junk additives.

Chocolate is made from the beans of the cacao tree, Theobroma CacaoPlant. Cacao is full of flavonoids that are commonly known for their antioxidant activity. A small bar of dark chocolate can contain as many flavonoids as six apples, four and a half cups of tea, or two glasses of red wine.

Properly processed dark chocolate actually provides great benefits without the unhealthy ingredients that are often included in the common milk chocolate bar. Good dark chocolate can serve as an appetite suppressant; lower your blood pressure, improve your mood, and add antioxidants.

The reason: Dark chocolate's bitter taste might help the body regulate appetite, or its higher amount of cocoa butter (it has stearic acid, which can slow digestion) may make the stomach stay full longer.

Some other great things about chocolate:

* Cacao, the source of chocolate, contains antibacterial agents that fight tooth decay. Of course, this is counteracted by the high sugar content of milk chocolate.
* The smell of chocolate may increase theta brain waves, resulting in relaxation.
* Chocolate contains phenylethylamine, a mild mood elevator.
* The cocoa butter in chocolate contains oleic acid, a mono-unsaturated fat, which may raise good cholesterol.
* The flavonoids in chocolate may help keep blood vessels elastic.
* Chocolate increases antioxidant levels in the blood.
* The carbohydrates in chocolate raise serotonin levels in the brain, resulting in a sense of well-being.

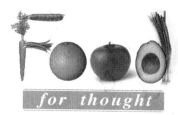

*for thought*

*To control a sweet tooth, simply have one or two small squares of dark chocolate after a meal. Because of the rich flavor of dark chocolate, that amount is enough to satisfy a sweet tooth while allowing you to consume very minimal calories (usually under 50 calories if the squares are small). In addition, you also get some antioxidant benefits, appetite satisfying benefits from the healthy fats, and MUCH less sugar than in most other desserts!*

Although dark chocolate has many great benefits, go easy because chocolate is high in calories, sugar and often other additives. Save it as a special treat and just eat a small amount of it at a time. If you get migraines, be aware that chocolate could be triggering them so exercise caution here.

# 24 Green Tea and Other Teas

*Is green tea good for weight loss?*

There has been heavy marketing in recent years for supplements containing either green tea or oolong tea (sometimes marketed under names as Wulong® or Wu-yi tea) and claiming to be a miracle weight-loss aid.

The truth is that green tea, white tea, oolong tea, and black tea (all types of teas originating from the same plant – the Camellia Sinensis plant) provide some minor benefits in the fat-burning process. However, the evidence appears that the fat-burning or metabolism-boosting effect is fairly small, and most supplements containing these teas are overhyped.

However, that doesn't mean there aren't big time benefits to these teas, including some small amount of benefit in the weight-loss department – just realize that teas are best in their naturally brewed form, and you don't need to buy expensive supplements containing tea extracts.

Green tea has received the most attention of all of the Camellia Sinensis plant teas. What is it about green tea? Well, the benefits of green tea are numerous. In fact, if you were to go to PubMed.com and do a search for green tea, you'd find over 2,000 studies performed on green tea and its components. Suddenly everyone is paying attention to green tea! Possible benefits are being investigated for weight loss, cancer prevention, antioxidant activity, cognitive enhancement, general good health and well being... and the list goes on and on.

### But why is green tea a possible aid for fat loss?

Many reasons. First of all, green tea is a source of caffeine, and delivered in a more mellow, sustained way than the caffeine jolt of coffee. Caffeine, of course, is a decent fat burner with a well-established track record. Green tea also slightly helps aid weight loss by increasing the metabolic rate, causing those who use it to experience a small increase in calorie burn (American Journal of Clinical Nutrition).

That makes it a decent quality fat burner in and of itself.

If that's all green tea did, this would be a pretty short section. Luckily, it provides additional benefits -- far and beyond what plain caffeine could do. First, it's a powerful anti-oxidant. Yes, just like Vitamin C and beta-carotene, and fruits and veggies! But researchers have suggested that the active ingredient (called epigallocatechin gallate) may be up to 200 times more powerful than Vitamin E as an antioxidant.

The best part is, green tea may be useful as a glucose regulator - meaning it slows the rise in blood sugar following a meal. When you keep your blood sugar stable, you cut down on your insulin response...that, in turn, means more controlled appetite and less stored fat!

It does this by slowing the action of a particular digestive enzyme called amylase. This enzyme is pivotal in the breakdown of starches (carbs) that can cause blood sugar levels to soar following a meal.

This is pretty exciting stuff - green tea might be a missing link in proper glucose management.

A recent study also validates green tea's effectiveness. Published in the American Journal of Clinical Nutrition, it indicated the ingestion of a tea rich in catechins leads to both a lowering of body fat AND of cholesterol levels. That is phenomenal news.

Additionally, green tea may inhibit fatty acid synthase. Fatty acid synthase is an enzymatic system that is involved in the process of turning carbohydrates into fat. Early animal studies suggest the inhibition of fatty acid synthase can lead to weight loss.

*Aside from plain water, green tea is the healthiest possible drink you can have with your meals or during the day.*

If that weren't enough, there's also evidence that consuming green tea high in catechins reduces cardiovascular risks..

In short, green tea's weight-loss benefits are a result of several mechanisms, including increased metabolism, a positive effect on blood sugar and insulin regulation, and the inhibition of certain enzymes, which are required for the processing of carbohydrates and fats. It also has been shown to lower LDL levels (that's the "bad" cholesterol) as well as triglyceride levels.

Best benefits start with two to three cups of tea a day. Not into hot liquids? Make some up and pour it over ice with a little stevia to sweeten it up. There are many types of green tea out there to choose from. Some have caffeine, some do not. Some are flavored with orange, chai, jasmine, etc. Look for a reputable brand and choose organic when possible.

Remember that white tea, oolong tea, and black tea are all from the same plant as green tea and may have similar benefits, but have simply been studied less than green tea. Each type of tea has unique antioxidants, so there may be additional benefits to mixing up your variety of teas.

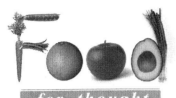

*Try this delicious iced tea mixture. Use some green tea bags, some white tea bags, and some oolong tea bags and make a mixed iced tea, sweetened just ever so lightly with a little stevia. For an herbal tea, try Celestial Seasonings® Berry Zinger tea over ice for a delicious refreshing summer drink.*

In addition, many herbal teas offer a huge variety of antioxidants and are a great substitute for sodas, juice, etc., which add empty calories and lead to weight gain. There are berry teas, red teas (a.k.a - rooibos tea), mint teas, chamomile teas, yerba mate, hibiscus teas, and others. All of these teas have additional unique antioxidants and individual benefits.

For example, hibiscus teas (the tea most commonly called "herbal tea") have been found in studies to help reduce blood pressure. Also, chamomile tea is known for its calming benefits and contains unique phytonutrients that can help to fight the effect of estrogenic pollutants or pesticides inside your body. All of these taste delicious hot or cold, and some are so good and naturally sweet (with 0 calories) they don't need anything else.

# 25 Stocking Your Kitchen

## *The Best Veggies and Fruits*

First, buy local whenever you can. Depending on where you live and what season it is, you may have a bounty of fresh fruits and vegetables grown near you. Many can be purchased at your local farmer's market, and some grocery stores now even carry local produce.

Benefits: You support your smaller, local farmer; the produce is infinitely more fresh than the kind you get at chain grocery stores that has been shipped for thousands of miles across the country or from other countries; and local produce generally is either organic or has less pesticides, herbicides and preservatives on them because it does not come from a huge factory farm - making them far, far healthier for you.

If you can't find or afford organic, or locally grown, then take a look at this list of non-organic foods to avoid. These foods are the most highly sprayed, commercially sold produce. So, if you can't get local or organic, try to avoid these in conventional form. They are laden with pesticides and toxins.

**The "Dirty Dozen"**

* Apples
* Cherries
* Grapes, imported (Chile)
* Nectarines
* Peaches
* Pears
* Raspberries
* Strawberries
* Bell peppers
* Celery
* Potatoes
* Spinach

The following fruits and veggies are much safer to eat in conventional form without having to pay extra for organic:

* Bananas
* Kiwi
* Mangos
* Papaya
* Pineapples
* Asparagus
* Avocado
* Broccoli
* Cauliflower
* Onions

## Why does organic cost more?

Growing organic food is more labor-intensive. And even though organic food is a growing industry, it doesn't have the economies of scale or government subsidies available to conventional growers. So if you have to buy conventional, follow these precautions to protect yourself from pesticides:

Buy fresh vegetables and fruits in season. When long storage and long-distance shipping are not required, fewer pesticides are used.

Trim tops and the very outer portions of celery, lettuce, cabbages, and other leafy vegetables that may contain the bulk of pesticide residues.

Peel and cook when appropriate, even though some nutrients and fiber are lost in the process.

Eat a wide variety of fruits and vegetables. This would limit exposure to any one type of pesticide residue.

Purchase only fruits and vegetables that are subject to USDA regulations. Produce imported from other countries is not grown under the same regulations as enforced by the USDA. We import a lot of produce from Mexico, and it is best to avoid unless it is organic.

Wait until just before preparation to wash or immerse your produce in clean water. When appropriate, scrub with a brush. This removes insect residue and dirt, as well as bacteria and some pesticide residues.

Special soaps or washes are not needed and could be harmful to you, depending on their ingredients. Cool water is perfectly fine.

## Other Stuff to Stock in Your Kitchen

O.K., now you know what you need to transform your kitchen and your body. There are many other foods, spices and condiments that also add to your healthy kitchen.

Basically, it all starts with making smart choices and avoiding temptations when you make your grocery store trip. Once you realize the reasons to avoid the junk and eat the good stuff, you get into some healthier habits. A lean, strong, healthy body will be the result, along with oodles of energy and a new outlook on life.

Let's start with stuff to keep on hand in your refrigerator. One or two times a week, load up on fresh veggies. During the summer, visit your local farmers' market frequently and get the freshest, tastiest produce on the planet. Outside of that, stock up on the produce at the grocery store.

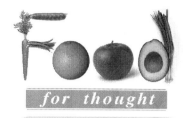

*for thought*

*Remember, if you don't have junk around the house, you're less likely to eat junk. If all you have is healthy food around the house, you're forced to make smart choices.*

# SHOPPING LIST

## *Start here:*

**Vegetables** like zucchini, onions, fresh mushrooms, spinach, broccoli, red peppers, cilantro, etc., to add to omelets, salads, stir-fry, shish kabobs, etc.

**Coconut milk** is a versatile staple to keep on hand. It can be used to mix in with smoothies, oatmeal or yogurt for a rich, creamy taste. Not only does coconut milk add a rich, creamy taste to lots of dishes, but it's also full of healthy, saturated fats such as medium chain triglycerides.

**Cottage cheese, ricotta cheese and yogurt** – Try cottage or ricotta cheese and yogurt together with chopped nuts and berries for a great mid-morning or mid-afternoon meal. Raw cheese (grass fed is the best) is awesome and a rich source of more useable calcium, Vitamin K2 for your bones and tons of enzymes.

**Almonds, pecans, walnuts, pistachios**—Chopped or whole, these are delicious and great sources of healthy fats. Grab a handful for a healthy, filling snack or throw some into your smoothies, salads and veggies.

**Whole eggs** – One of nature's richest sources of nutrients (and remember, they increase your GOOD cholesterol so stop fearing them). Get them free-range if at all possible. Always include the yolks - the richest source of nutrients in the egg.

*Nut butters* – Peanut butter is a bit boring, so get creative and try almond butter, cashew butter, or even macadamia butter...delicious and unbeatable nutrition!

*Salsa* – Get creative and try some of the exotic varieties of salsas. Lots of grocery stores now sell this in the fresh produce aisle, and it is as delicious and fresh tasting as homemade. Try this on your eggs in the morning for a great healthy eye-opener!

*Butter* – Don't believe the naysayers; butter, especially from grass-fed cows, adds great flavor to anything and can be part of a healthy diet (just keep the quantity small because it is calorie dense). NEVER use margarine, unless you want to assure yourself of a heart attack.

*Avocados* –Awesome taste...plus a great source of healthy fats, fiber, and other nutrients. Try adding them to wraps, salads, on top of omelets, or in sandwiches.

*Whole grain wraps or gluten-free brown rice wraps and bread* - Look for wraps and bread with at least four to five grams of fiber per 20 grams of total carbs. Remember that it's best to minimize grain intake if fat loss is your goal, so use these sparingly.

*Greens* – Stock up weekly on baby greens, dark green leaf lettuce or red leaf lettuce, romaine, arugula, and organic baby spinach to top sandwiches, throw into "green" smoothies, and for salads with dinner.

*Home-made salad dressing* – Use balsamic vinegar, Udo's Choice® Oil Blend, and extra virgin olive oil. This is much better than store bought salad dressings, which mostly use highly-refined soybean oil (full of inflammation-causing free radicals). Try this mix: olive oil, balsamic vinegar, chopped fresh basil and thyme, garlic, salt and pepper. Anything you pour this dressing over will really taste terrific!

*Fresh herbs* - Basil, thyme, oregano, cilantro – chop and toss on salads, throw into eggs, and garnish meat dishes.

## *Staples for the freezer:*

*Frozen fish* – Keep it wild! Try different kinds of fish each week. There are so many varieties out there you never have to get bored. Trader Joe's is a great place to find wild-caught frozen fish of all kinds.

*Frozen berries* – During the local growing season buy fresh, but during the rest of the year, keep a supply of frozen blueberries, raspberries, blackberries, strawberries, cherries, etc. to add to high fiber cereal, oatmeal, cottage cheese, yogurt, or smoothies.

*Frozen veggies* – Again, when the growing season is over and you can no longer get local fresh produce, frozen veggies are the best option, since they often have higher nutrient contents - even compared to fresh produce that has been shipped across the country. Or buy lots of the fresh veggies when they are available locally and freeze in small portions.

*Frozen chicken breasts* – Free-range, if at all possible. Very convenient to cook up for a quick addition to wraps or sliced on top of a salad for a quick meal.

*Frozen grass-fed meats* – Bison, beef, lamb, goat, etc.

## *Staples for the pantry:*

*Oat bran and steel cut oats* – Higher fiber than those little packs of instant oats that are full of sugar and high on the glycemic index.

*Cans of coconut milk* – To be transferred to a container in the fridge after opening.

*Various antioxidant rich teas* – Green, oolong, white, and rooibos are some of the best.

*Variety of herb teas* – Drink hot or cold, sweeten with a touch of honey or stevia if necessary. Have fun trying different flavors!

*Stevia* – The best natural, non-caloric sweetener. Read more at http://Naturally-Stevia.com

*Organic maple syrup and agave nectar*– Stay away from the commercial syrups that are basically unhealthy, high-fructose corn syrup...only real maple syrup can be considered real food. Try a small amount over oatmeal, or added to your post workout shake for muscle-glycogen replenishing carbs.

*Raw honey* – Even better than processed honey, it contains higher quantities of beneficial nutrients and lots of enzymes. Honey has even been proven in studies to improve glucose metabolism (how you process carbs).Try a teaspoon or so in your tea. Yes, it is pure sugar, but it does have some nutritional benefits, and a teaspoon of honey is only five grams of carbs.

*Whole wheat or brown rice pasta* – Much higher fiber than normal pastas, brown rice pasta can usually be found in the gluten-free section of the grocery store or health food store, and it is delicious. Even if you don't have a gluten allergy, its best to limit the wheat that you eat; many people may have problems digesting wheat and gluten and not even be aware. Remember that if fat loss is your goal, we recommend limiting your grain intake, so keep any pastas as only a once a week cheat meal.

*Brown rice and other higher-fiber rice* – NEVER eat white rice! You can purchase the slow-cooking brown rice variety in bags, or buy instant or frozen. A delicious, nutty brown rice to try is from Trader Joe's, and comes pre-cooked and frozen.

*Cans of black or pinto beans* – Add to Mexican wraps for the fiber and high nutrition content. Also, beans are surprisingly one of the best sources of youth promoting antioxidants! These are also good thrown into salsas for more protein and fiber.

*Tomato sauces* – A great source of lycopene! Watch out for the brands that are loaded with high-fructose corn syrup. Your best and cheapest bet is to stock up on organic tomato sauce and make your own Italian sauce seasoning with salt, pepper, oregano, basil, garlic, and whatever else you feel like throwing in!

Or you can always load up on in-season, organic tomatoes from your farmers' market, can them, and prepare your tomato sauce as you need it throughout the rest of the year!

*Dark chocolate (as dark as possible)* – A favorite treat that satisfies sweets cravings, plus provides loads of antioxidants at the same time. It's still calorie dense, so keep to just a couple squares.

*Organic unsweetened cocoa powder* – Mix this into a smoothie for an extra jolt of antioxidants, or make your own low-sugar hot cocoa by mixing cocoa powder into hot milk with stevia and a couple of melted dark chocolate chunks.

*Sea Salt* – Lots of grocery stores now carry sea salt, and a fun one to try is the kind you can grind yourself. Nothing tastes better than freshly ground sea salt on your healthy food (Yes! There is a huge difference!) And sea salt is loaded with minerals like magnesium and potassium, and is not nearly as bad for those with reactive high blood pressure. A little goes a long way.

# BUYING GUIDE

*Grass-fed beef, bison, veal, lamb, goat, free-range chicken, grass-fed raw cheeses, grass-fed butter and more* - The best source of high quality grass-fed meat, grass-fed raw cheese, grass-fed butter, free-range chicken, humanely raised pork, wild-caught fish, nutraceuticals, organic nuts, snacks, and more is U.S. Wellness Meats at **http://healthygrassfed.2ya.com.**

This company ships across the country, and in most places you will receive your order at your door in two days. Meat comes vacuum packed and frozen in insulated cold cartons, unless ordered fresh. The is some of the best tasting meat you will ever have! This company cannot be beat for high quality, grass-fed meats, cheese and snacks. U.S. Wellness Meats also carries a great low sugar, high-fructose-corn-syrup-free sports water that fuels active lifestyles.

*Wild Caught Fish* - Best online source for a great variety of delicious, wild-caught sustainable salmon and high omega-3, certified pure, sushi-grade fresh and frozen fish is Vital Choice Seafood: **http://www.vitalchoice.com/index.cfm.** Check out the tabs "Doctors Top Choices" and "Product Starter Packs" for great ideas on what to order. Also try Alaskan Sablefish for a rich, delicious, melt-in-your-mouth, super healthy, high omega-3 treat. Trader Joe's is also a great place to buy small packages of wild-caught frozen fish of various kinds, as is your local grocery store. Look for "wild-caught" not "farm-raised."

*Nuts* - Obviously the grocery does carry nuts, but try to find the raw nuts, or those without added omega-6 oils, which kind of defeat the purpose of eating them. One of the best places to find great selections of nuts, trail mix, etc. at great prices is Trader Joe's.

*Raw Milk* -Go to **http://www.realmilk.com/where1.html.** Find your state and click on it to search for dairy farms near you. Some farms will ship to your home, or deliver close to where you live. Some of these farms also carry free-range organic eggs, grass-fed meats, and other items as well.

*Stevia* - is now readily available at most grocery stores. The more pure version of stevia is usually sold in health-food sections of grocery stores or healthier food stores like Trader Joe's and Whole Foods. Lots of times stevia is placed in the "supplement" aisle, because of FDA rulings. Expect to see stevia or derivatives of stevia in mainstream soft drinks, frozen treats, and other low calorie sweetened items. That still doesn't mean these are great items to be ingesting, but possibly less unhealthy than before!

*Gluten-free brown rice pasta and gluten-free brown rice wrap*s- Grocery stores are really starting to pick up on the gluten-free trend, so many actually may have a gluten-free section in the store. Otherwise check your regular pasta aisle for brown rice or whole wheat pasta. Trader Joe's and Whole Foods have a big variety of gluten-free brown rice pastas of all different shapes and sizes.

*Sea Salt* - Most grocery stores now carry the rock sea salt in the little grinder. Rather than buy a new grinder with salt in it every time, you can buy a bigger container of sea salt in the larger crystal size and just fill up the grinder. It saves money and keeps you stocked with great tasting salt.

*Dark chocolate* - Healthier food stores carry great dark chocolate, but many grocery stores now carry decent dark chocolate as well. Remember that milk chocolate is more fattening, contains more sugar, and is not as good for you, so stick with dark chocolate that is at least 70 percent cocoa, with no additives or preservatives.

*Coconut oil* - Whole Foods or your health food store will have it. Your grocery store may also have it in the health foods aisle. Be sure it is in its natural state, and not hydrogenated.

*Healthy energy bars* - Try Whole Foods, Trader Joes, your local grocery store's health food aisle, or order online.

# 26 Begin the Transformation

S
o there you have it. Remove the offensive, empty-calorie processed foods and replace them with real, nutrient-dense foods, and your body will be transformed from a fat factory to a fat-burning, lean machine. The transformation may not happen overnight, so give it time. But it WILL happen! And in the process, you may find that you no longer want to eat junk food. Nourishing your body with healthy, nutritious REAL food will satisfy hunger and give your body what it needs. You will begin to like how you feel – and look – and you will not crave junk food.

If you generally purchase and eat the foods listed in this book, you will not only begin to change your eating habits for good, but you will change into a lean, strong, energetic, younger-looking you. You will probably also notice some other great benefits to this diet transformation too: shinier, thicker hair, clearer skin, less sinus problems, less colds and flu, better sex drive, more energy, and quicker recovery time when you work out—to name just a few things. Mentally you should feel sharper, clearer, happier and less irritable too.

I know it isn't realistic to think that you will eat ONLY the foods on this list, but taking smart snacks with you when you are on the run and choosing healthy menu items when dining out should keep you on track. And don't despair if you deviate or have a day when you end up eating poorly. Just get back on track again the next day. A general rule of thumb is to try to eat healthy ninety percent of the time and don't beat yourself up for that other ten percent!

Just remember these simple guidelines:

* Eat foods that are minimally processed or not processed at all.
* Avoid as much as possible any food that comes in a package with
    an ingredient list of more than three or four items.
* Eat food that is as close to the way Mother Nature created it as you can.
* Give your body the fuel it needs and the fat will melt away.

Choose the apple over the packaged applesauce. Eat raw nuts, not the sugar coated, hydrogenated, salty kind from the can. Pick up the raw unpasteurized cheese to nibble on, not the processed stuff in a squirt can. Eat the meat that was raised the way nature intended—grass-fed, free-range or wild-caught. Eat good fats—the ones that occur naturally in foods, not the processed vegetable oils or trans fats.

Change your shopping habits. Buy local and hit the farmers' markets when you can, shop at healthy grocery stores like Whole Foods or Trader Joe's or the local "mom and pop" health food store. If you have to go to the regular grocery store, try to shop only the perimeter of the store. Most of the inner aisles of the store are full of shelves lined with processed and packaged foods. No need to be tempted.

### *Good luck with your transformation!*

Enjoy your lean body and glowing health!

Your friends will all wonder what your secret to success is, and when they ask, share this book with them. You may help change a life!

# REFERENCES

## Health in the U.S.

Keehan, S. et al. "Health Spending Projections Through 2017, Health Affairs Web Exclusive W146: 21 February 2008.

California Health Care Foundation. Health Care Costs 101 -- 2005. 02 March 2005.

Mokdad AH, Marks JS, Stroup DF, Gerberding JL. Actual causes of death in the United States, 2000. JAMA. 2004;291 :1238—1245.

Stampfer MJ, Hu FB, Manson JE, et al. Primary prevention of coronary heart disease in women through diet and lifestyle. N Engl J Med. 2000;343:16—22.

Knoops KT, de Grrot LC, Kromhout D, et al. Mediterranean diet, lifestyle factors, and 10-year mortality in elderly European men and women: the HALE project. JAMA. 2004;292(12):1433—1439.

Chiuve SE, McCullough ML, Sacks FM, Rimm EB. Healthy lifestyle factors in the primary prevention of coronary heart disease among men (Benefits among users and nonusers of lipid-lowering and antihypertensive medications). Circulation. 2006; 114(2): 160—167. CrossRef

Kurth T, Moore SC, Gaziano M, et al. Healthy lifestyle and the risk of stroke in women. Arch Intern Med. 2006;166(13):1403—1409.

Esposito K, Pontillo A, Di Palo C, et al. Effect of weight loss and lifestyle changes on vascular inflammatory markers in obese women: a randomized trial. JAMA. 2003;289(14):1799—1804.

American College of Sports Medicine position stand. Exercise for patients with coronary artery disease. Med Sci Sports Exerc. 1 994;26(3) :i—vhttp ://www.ms-se.com/pt/pt-core/tem plate-journal! msse/media/0394.pdfAccessed October 13, 2008.

Subar AF, Thompson FE, Kipnis V, et al. Comparative validation of the Block, Willett, and National Cancer Institute food frequency questionnaires: the Eating at America's Table Study. Am J Epidemiol. 2001 ;1 54:1089—1099a.

Mokdad AH, Ford ES, Bowman BA, et al. Prevalence of obesity, diabetes, and obesity-related health risk factors, 2001. JAMA. 2003 ;289:76—79.

Expert Panel on Detection, Evaluation, and Treatment of High Blood Cholesterol in Adults. Executive Summary of the Third Report of the National Cholesterol Education Program (NCEP) Expert Panel on Detection, Evaluation, and Treatment of High Blood Cholesterol in Adults (Adult Treatment Panel III). JAMA. 2001 ;285:2486—2497.

Zhang C, Rexrode KM, van Dam RM, et al. Abdominal obesity and the risk of all-cause, cardiovascular, and cancer mortality: sixteen years of follow-up in US women. Circulation. 2008;117(13):1 658—1667.

Katzmarzyk PT, Janssen I, Ardern CI. Physical inactivity, excess adiposity and premature mortality. Obes Rev. 2003 ;4(4):257—290.

Strine TW, Mokdad AH, Dube SR, et al. The association of depression and anxiety with obesity and unhealthy behaviors among community-dwelling US adults. Gen Hosp Psychiatry. 2008;30(2):127—137.

Mosca L, McGillen C, Rubenfire M. Gender differences in barriers to lifestyle change for cardiovascular disease prevention. J Womens Health. 1998;7(6):711—715.

Mainous AG, Baker R, Koopman RJ, et al. Impact of the population at risk of diabetes on projections of diabetes burden in the United States: an epidemic on the way. Diabetologia. 2007 ;50(5):903—905.

Kahn R, Robertson RM, Smith R, Eddy D. The impact of prevention on reducing the burden of cardiovascular disease. Diabetes Care. 2008;3 1(8): 1686—1696.

Bibbins-Domingo K, Coxson P, Pletcher Mi, et al. Adolescent overweight and future adult coronary heart disease. N Engl I Med. 2007;357:2371 —2379.

Childhood Obesity Prevention Study, Institute of Medicine of the National Academies, September 2004; drawn from Preventing Childhood Obesity: Health in the Balance, 2005, Institute of Medicine, www.iom.edu

Sydney Morning Herald, "Crime, punishment, and a Junk Food Diet," http://www.smh.com.au/ articles/2006/1 1/15/11 63266639865.html

cnn.com, http://www.cnn.com/2007/H EALTH/diet.fitness/09/22/kd.g upta.column/index.html

www.eduplace.com

## The Low-Fat I High Obesity Diet

A Literature Review of the Value-Added Nutrients found in Grass-fed Beef Products. C.A. Daley(1), A.Abbott(1), P. Doyle(1), G. Nader(2), and S. Larson(2). College of Agriculture, California State University, Chico(1). University of California Cooperative Extension Service(2)

Conjugated linoleic acid reduces body fat mass in overweight and obese humans. Blankson H, Stakkstand i, Fagertun H, Thorn E, Wadstein I, Gudmundson 0.1 Nutr. 2000; 130:2943-48. French P, Stanton C, Lawless F, O'Riordan EG, Monahan Fi, Caffrey P1, Moloney. Fatty acid composition, including conjugated linoleic acid of intramuscular fat from steers offered grazed grass, grass silage or concentrate-based diets. AP, 2000. 1. Anim. Sci. 78:2849-2855.

Lonn EM, Yusuf S. Is there a role for antioxidant vitamins in the prevention of cardiovascular diseases? An update on epidemiological and clinical trials data. Can I Cardiol 1997;13:957-65.

Yang A, Brewster Mi, Lanari MC, Tume RK. Effect of vitamin E supplementation on a-tocopherol and B-carotene concentrations in tissues from pasture and grain-fed cattle. Meat Science 2002a; 60(1):35-40.

## The Core Nutrition

Cordain L, Eaton SB, Sebastian A, Mann N, Lindeberg S, Watkins BA, O'Keefe JH, Brand-Miller J. Origins and evolution of the Western diet: health implications for the 21st century. Am J Clin Nutr. 2005 Feb;81 (2):341 -54.

# The Advanced Nutrition

J Am Coll Cardiol 2004;43:731-3

Dr. Ron Rosedale, author, The Rosedale Diet, www.DiabetesHealth.com

Cordain L, Eades MR, Eades MD. Hyperinsulinemic diseases of civilization: more than just syndrome X. Comp Biochem Physiol Part A 2003;136:95-112.

New Scientist, 1 September 2001

Osterdahi M, Kocturk T, Koochek A, Wändell PE. Effects of a short—term intervention with a paleolithic diet in healthy volunteers. Eur J Clin Nutr. 2008 May;62(5):682-5.

Lindeberg 5, Jönsson T, Granfeldt Y, Borgstrand E, Soffman J, Sjöström K, Ahrén B. A Palaeolithic diet improves glucose tolerance more than a Mediterranean-like diet in individuals with ischaemic heart disease. Diabetologia. 2007 Sep;50(9):1795-807.

Jönsson T, Ahrén B, Pacini G, Sundler F, Wierup N, Steen 5, Sjoberg T, Ugander M, Frostegrd J, Göransson L, Lindeberg S. A Paleolithic diet confers higher insulin sensitivity, lower C-reactive protein and lower blood pressure than a cereal-based diet in domestic pigs. Nutr Metab (Lond). 2006 Nov 2;3:39.

Westerterp-Plantenga MS, Rolland V, Wilson SM, Westerterp KR. Satiety related to 24-h diet- induced thermogenesis during high protein/carbohydrate vs high fat diets measured in a respiratory chamber. Eur J Clin Nutr. 1999;53:495-502.

Feinman RD, Fine EJ. Thermodynamics and metabolic advantage of weight loss diets. Metab Syndr Relat Disord. 2003;1 :209-19.

O'Keefe JH Jr, Cordain L. Cardiovascular disease resulting from a diet and lifestyle at odds with our Paleolithic genome: how to become a 21st-century hunter-gatherer. Mayo Clin Proc. 2004 Jan;79(1):101-8.

Cordain L. The nutritional characteristics of a contemporary diet based upon Paleolithic food groups. J Am Nutraceut Assoc 2002; 5:1 5-24.

Cordain L. Syndrome X: Just the tip of the hyperinsulinemia iceberg. Medikament 2001; 6:46-51.

## Meal Ideas Core and Advanced Nutrition

Layman DK, Evans EM, Erickson D, Seyler J, Weber J, Bagshaw D, Griel A, Psota I, Kris-Etherton P. A Moderate-Protein Diet Produces Sustained Weight Loss and Long-Term Changes in Body Composition and Blood Lipids in Obese Adults. J. Nutr. 139: 514-521, 2009.

Weigle DS, Breen PA, Matthys CC, Callahan HS, Meeuws KE, Burden VR, Purnell JG. A high-protein diet induces sustained reductions in appetite, ad libitum caloric intake, and body weight despite compensatory changes in diurnal plasma leptin and ghrelin concentrations. Am J Clin Nutr. 2005;82:41 -8.

The Leptin Diet by Byron J. Richards.

## Special Focus: Water

Epidemiology 1998;9(1):21-28, 29-35

Consumer Reports: "Is Your Water Safe to Drink?"

An Analysis of the Causes of Tooth Decay, Professor Cornelius Steeling, Department of Chemistry, University of Arizona

John Curnette, et al, "Fluoride-mediated Activation of the Respiratory burst in Human Neutrophils," Journal of Clinical Investigation, Vol. 63, pp. 637-657 (1979)

International Bottled Water Association (IBWA)

Dr. Theodore Baroody, "Alkalize or Die"

## Special Focus: Pesticides

The Environmental Working Group, www.foodnews.org or www.ewg.org

## Special Focus:Sugar

Skov AR, Toubro 5, Ronn B, Holm L, Astrup A. Randomized trial on protein versus carbohydrate in ad libitum fat reduced diet for the treatment of obesity. IntJ Obes Relat Metab Disord. 1 999;23 :528-3 6.

Life Without Bread by Christian Allan, PhD and Wolfgang Lutz, M.D. Do National Dietary Guidelines Do More Harm Than Good? Science Daily
McKinney, Dr. Neil, Vital Victoria Naturopathic Clinic, Ltd. Sugar feeds cancer. www.drneilmckinney.ca

## Special Focus: Dairy

Cows' milk fat components as potential anticarcinogenic agents. Parodi PW. J Nutr 1997; 127:1055-1060.

Lancet, Ohio Agricultural Experiment, Annual Review of Biochemistry, Newman and Deutsch, Kim Work. Archives of Pediatrics & Adolescent Medicine June 2005;159(6):543-550

www.realmilk.com

Thomas Cohen , Sally Fallon. "Fight the Pasteurization Myth." Weston A. Price Foundation WiseTraditions.1999. Weston A. Price Foundation. 10 June 2009 http://www.westonaprice.org/basicnutrition/vitamin-k2.html

Lipinski, Lori. "Milk: It Does a Body Good? It all depends on where it comes from, doesn't it?." Wise Traditions in Food, Farming and the Healing Arts, the quarterly magazine of the Weston A. Price Foundation. April 2003. Weston A. Price Foundation. 5/ 07/2009. http://www.westonaprice.org/transition/dairy.html

Jonsson, Randolph. Raw-milk-facts.com. 2004. White Tiger construction. 06 07 2009. http://www.raw-milk-facts.com/
Gates , Donna. "The 20 health benefits of real butter." Body Ecology Diet. 2009. Bodyecology.com. 02/06/09. http://www.bodyecology.com/07/07/05/benefits_of_real_butter.php

The Scientific Committee on Veterinary Measures Relating to Public Health. "Assessment of Potential Risks to Human Health from Hormone Residues in Bovine Meat and Meat Products." European Commission, April 30, 1999.
http://www.sustainabletable.org/issues/hormones/

## Special Focus: Coconut

Kaunitz H, Dayrit CS. Coconut oil consumption and coronary heart disease. Philippine Journal of Internal Medicine 1992;30:165-171. Prior IA, Davidson F, Salmond CE, Czochanska Z. Cholesterol, coconuts, and diet on Polynesian atolls: a natural experiment: the Pukapuka and Tokelau Island studies. American Journal of Clinical Nutrition 1981 ;34:1552—1561.

Kurup PA, Rajmohan T. II. Consumption of coconut oil and coconut kernel and the incidence of atherosclerosis. Coconut and Coconut Oil in Human Nutrition, Proceedings. Symposium on Coconut and Coconut Oil in Human Nutrition. 27 March 1994. Coconut Development Board, Kochi, India, 1995, pp 35-59

New York Times, Medical Science, Tuesday, January 29, 1991. Common virus seen as having early role in arteries' clogging (byline Sandra Blakeslee).

Coconut: In Support of good Health in the 21st Century, by Mary 0. Enig, Ph.D., F.A.C.N. Coconut Oil Miracle, by Bruce Fife, C.N, N.D

Enig, Mary, Ph.D., and Fallon, Sally. The Oiling of America. Nexus Magazine, December 1998-January 1999 and February 1999-March 1999.

Mercier, Y., P. Gatellier, M. Renerre (2004). "Lipid and protein oxidation in vitro, and antioxidant potential in meat from Charolais cows finished on pasture or mixed diet." Meat Science 66: 467- 473.

## Special Focus: Nuts

"Health Benefits of Nuts, the Snack that Benefits Your Health."The Healthier Life. August 2003.

Agora Lifestyles. 05/05/09 http://www.thehealthierlife.co.uk/natural-healtharticles/
nutrition/health-benefits-of-nuts-00841.html

# Special Focus: Toxins

Starr Hull, Dr. Janet. Aspartame Dangers Revealed. 2006. Dr. Janet Starr Hull. 10 June 2009. http://www.sweetpoison.com/

"Nowhere to Hide" Persistent Toxic Chemicals in the U.S. Food Supply, Mar 2001, Pesticide Action Network North America.

Type 2 diabetes May be Linked to Pesticide Exposure. Environmental News Service, Cambridge, UK, January 25, 2008. http://www.ens-newswi re.com/ens/jan2008/2008-01 -25-04.asp

Ephraim, RD, CCN, Rebecca. "Aspartame: Diet-astrous Results." Wise Traditions in Food, Farming and the Healing Arts. 06 2000. Weston A. Price Foundation. 06/06/09. http://www.trit.us/modern-food/aspartame.html

Ellison, M.Sc., Shane. "Artificial Sweetner Explodes Internally." The People's Chemist. 2008. The People's Chemist.com 03/07/09. http://www.thepeopleschemist.com/view_learning.php?learning_id=14

# Special Focus: Animal Products

"The Welfare of Cattle in Beef Production; A Summary of the Scientific Evidence A Farm Sanctuary Report." Farm Santuary. 2009. 01 07 2009. http://www.farmsanctuary.org/mediacenter/beef_report.html

Stier , Ken. "Fish Farming's Growing Dangers." Time Magazine.19 09 2007. Time Magazine. May 15, 2009. http://www.time.com/time/health/article/0,8599,1663604,00.html

Extension Toxicology Network (EXTONET), University of Oregon, September, 1993. http://extoxnet.orst.edu/tibsfbioaccum.htm

Australian Academy of Science, NOVA Science in the News: The bitter-sweet taste of toxic substances: DDT and biological concentration. http:f/www.science.org.au/nova/index.htm. http://www.science.org.au/nova/036/O36box03.htm

Public health implications of meat production and consumption. Polly Walker, Pamela Rhubart-Berg, Shawn McKenzie, Kristin Kelling, Robert S Lawrence, Johns Hopkins Bloomberg School of Public Health. Public Health Nutrition: 8(4), 348—356 DOI: 10.1079/PHN2005727

"Food Democracy, Fish: Fresh vs. farmed, what you need to know." Food Democracy. May2008.http://fooddemocracy.wordpress. com/2008/05/20/fish-fresh-vs-farmed-what-you-needto-know/

Bell Muzaurieta, Annie. "Farmed Fish Might Be Unhealthy: New Research Shows Popular Farmed Fish Might Adversely Affect Your Heart Health." The Daily Green. May 2008. Hearst Communcia-tions. 07/15/09. http://www.thedailygreen.com/healthy-eating/eat-safe/farmedtilapia-health-effects-44071408#ixzz0LMdStrCV&C

## Special Focus: Pork and Shellfish

The New England Journal of Medicine April 27, 2000;342:1250-1253

Mayo Clin Proc December 1997;72:1133-1136,1197-1198

FDA Medical Bulletin, March 1993, p. 6.

Harvard Health Letter, June 1993

Thomas Arnold, MD, Medical Director, Louisiana Poison Control Center, Associate Professor and Chairman, Department of Emer-gency Medicine, Section of Clinical Toxicology, Louisiana State University Health Sciences Center

## Special Focus: Soy

Kaayla T. Daniel, Phd, CCN, author, The Whole Soy Story

## Special Focus: Corn

Mercola, Joseph. "Corn Caused Widespread Disease Among Some Native Americans." Mercola.com. March 06, 2000. http://articles. mercola.com/sites/articles/archive/2000/06/03/corn-part-one.aspx

## Special Focus: Raw vs. Cooked Food

Rauma AL, Törrönen R, Hnninen 0, Verhagen H, Mykknen H. Anti-oxidant status in long-term j adherents to a strict uncooked vegan diet. Department of Clinical Nutrition, University of Kuopio, Finland. PMID: 7491884: South Med J. 1985 Jul;78(7):841-4.

Douglass JM, Rasgon IM, Fleiss PM, Schmidt RD, Peters SN, Abel-mann EA. Effects of a raw food diet on hypertension and obesity. PMID: 4012382

Does Plastic in Microwave Pose Health Problems? Wall Street Journal, 12 Oct 1998. http://www. mindfully.org/Plastic/Microwave-Health-Problems.htm

Winston Craig, MPH, PhD, RD. "Health Benefits of Green Leafy Vegetables Greens - A Neglected Gold Mine." Vegetarianism and vegetarian nutrition. June 23 2009. http://citationmachine.net/index2.php?reqstyleid=1&reqsrcid=14&mode=form&more=&source_title=Web%20Document&source_mod=&stylename=MLA.

Masterjohn, Chris. "On the trail of the elusive X-factor." Weston A. Price Foundation WiseTraditions in Food, Farming and the Healing Arts. Spring, 2007. Weston A. PriceFoundation.06/10/ 09. http://www.westonaprice.org/basicnutrition/vitamin-k2.html

Ellison, M.Sc., Shane. "Fat for Energy and Raw Athletic Power."U.S. Wellness Meats Newsletter,September 15, 2007.U.S. Wellness Meats, 2007.05/13/09 http://www.uswellnessmeats.com/newsletter_archive/newsletter/2007/September_16_2007_Newsletter.html

Dolson, Laura. "Eat Your Greens!How to Cook Greens, Types of Greens, Recipes, Cooking Tips,." About.com. August 2008. About.com. 06/15/09http://lowcarbdiets.about.com/od/cooking/a/greensrecipes.htm

Dolson, Laura. "Green Leafy Vegetables - Nutritional Powerhous-es,." About.com. June2008.About.com, 06/15/09.http://lowcarbdiets.about.com/od/lowcarbsuperfoods/a/greensnutrition.htm

## Kitchen Clean Out

Reinhardt-Martin, Jane, RD. A summary of cooking and stability studies in flax seed. www.flaxrd. com

Ratnayake WMN, Behrens WA, Fischer PWF, ['Abbe MR, Mongeau R, and Beare-Rogers JL. "Flaxseed Chemical Stability and Nutritional Properties." Journal of Nutritional Biochemistry 3 (1992): 232— 240.

Chen Z-Y, Ratnayake WMN, and Cunnane SC. "Stability of Flaxseed during baking." Journal of American Oil Chemists Society 71(1992): 629-632.
National Statistics, London, England, 18 August 2006. www.statistics.gov.uk

Canadians spending more on eating out, 28 June 2006. www.statcan.gc.ca

Vitamins Ft Supplements

National Institute of Health Clinical Nutrition Center, 2002: Facts about dietary supplements: Vitamin A and Carotenoids.

Shaw, Jonathan. "The Deadliest Sin: From survival of the fittest to staying fit just to survive: scientists probe the benefits of exercise-- and the dangers of sloth." Harvard Magazine, March-April 2004: 36.

Willett, Walter C, and Meir J Stampfer. Review Offers Lowdown on Who Needs Vitamins (Reuters Health story on The New England Journal of Medicine 2001 ;345:1819-1824. January 2, 2002. http://preventdisease.com/news/articles/who_needs_vitamins.shtm I (accessed July 19, 2008)


# Taking Action

The American Journal of Medicine, Volume 122, Issue 6, Pages 528-534 (June 2009)

Traci Mann, A. Janet Tomiyama, Erika Westling, Ann-Marie Lew, Barbra Samuels, and Jason Chatman; University of California, Los Angeles April, 2007, American Psychologist, the journal of the American Psychological Association

The Fat Burning Kitchen:  Your 24-Hour Diet Transformation to Make Your Body a Fat-Burning Machine by Mike Geary - Certified Personal Trainer, Certified Nutrition  Specialist & Catherine Ebeling - RN, BSN

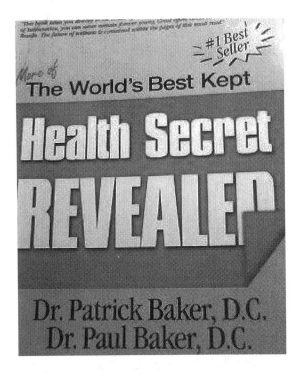

## The World's Best Kept Health Secret Revealed

Available at www.doctorspaulandpatrick.com

In this book, Dr. Patrick Baker, Dr. Paul Baker and other leading wellness Doctors of Chiropractic explore how to provide new levels of energy, health and wellness. They show ways to stop and reverse health challenges and make conscious choices that could transform your life and the lives of loved ones. These doctors provide you with information that could help you heal yourself and then, using what you have learned, help heal your family. Doctors of Chiropractic help the body naturally reverse current health problems and prevent future ones. Each year, over 30 million people choose this proven form of healthcare and wellness care.

Made in the USA
Charleston, SC
10 February 2012